SIMPLE
MEAL SOLUTIONS
for INSULIN RESISTANCE

SIMPLE MEAL SOLUTIONS
for INSULIN RESISTANCE

75 Recipes to Improve Insulin Resistance
and Support Stable Blood Sugar

Megan Koehn, RDN, LD

FAIR WINDS

Quarto.com

© 2025 Quarto Publishing Group USA Inc.
Text © 2025 Megan Koehn

First Published in 2025 by Fair Winds Press, an imprint of The Quarto Group,
100 Cummings Center, Suite 265-D, Beverly, MA 01915, USA.
T (978) 282-9590 F (978) 283-2742

Fair Winds Press titles are also available at discount for retail, wholesale, promotional, and bulk purchase. For details, contact the Special Sales Manager by email at specialsales@quarto.com or by mail at The Quarto Group, Attn: Special Sales Manager, 100 Cummings Center, Suite 265-D, Beverly, MA 01915, USA.

29 28 27 26 25   1 2 3 4 5

ISBN: 978-0-7603-9679-7

Digital edition published in 2025
eISBN: 978-0-7603-9680-3

Library of Congress Cataloging-in-Publication Data availble.

Design and Page Layout: Megan Jones Design
Cover Image: Wendi Washington-Hunt, wwhfoodphotography.com
Photography: Wendi Washington-Hunt, wwhfoodphotography.com

Printed in China

The information in this book is for educational purposes only. It is not intended to replace the advice of a physician or medical practitioner. Please see your health-care provider before beginning any new health program.

To my husband, Maxwell—my greatest supporter and Chief of Morale. Your unwavering belief in me has fueled my journey, pushing me to grow my company and help more people with insulin resistance and diabetes. I couldn't have done this without you.

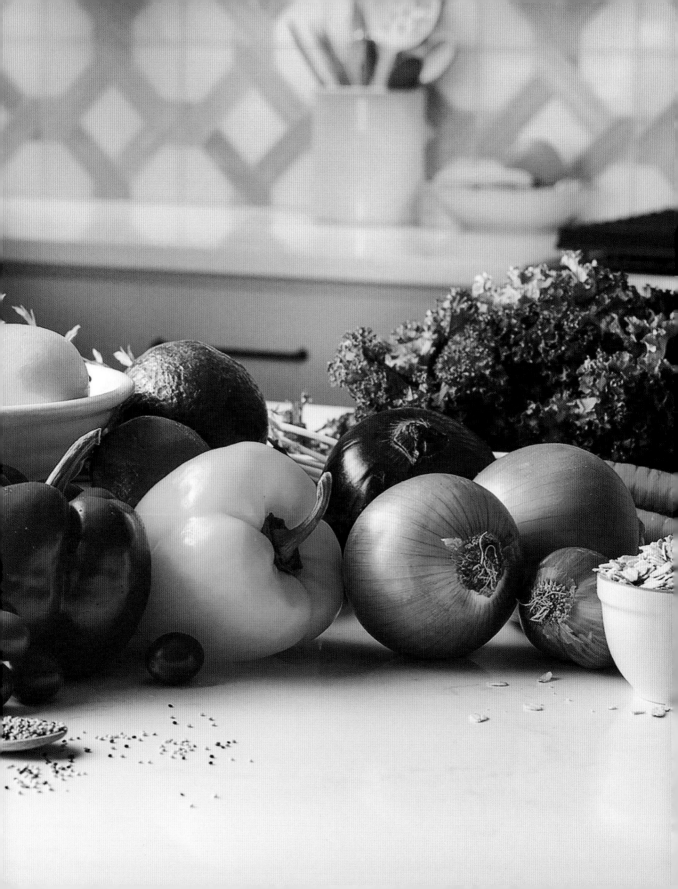

have to spend all your time cooking to meet your nutritional goals. I've also provided action steps for meal planning so you can easily adjust the recipes according to the number of people you're cooking for.

In my practice as an RDN, I never ask my clients to give up their favorite foods. Why? This helps them to manage insulin resistance without feeling like they are on a diet (no one likes feeling deprived!). Remember, there is no one-size-fits-all approach to healthy eating patterns, and no single diet works for everyone. For example, some people manage insulin resistance well with a vegan lifestyle, while others find this completely unsustainable. My goal is to help thousands more people succeed by taking a more individualized approach.

One final note: Each person is unique and so are their needs. For that reason, I recommend getting support in your health journey to ensure that you're working towards a sustainable approach and are assessing other lifestyle areas that are important when it comes to managing insulin resistance, such as physical activity, timing of meals and snacks, stress management, and mindfulness.

Ready to lower your insulin resistance? Let's get started!

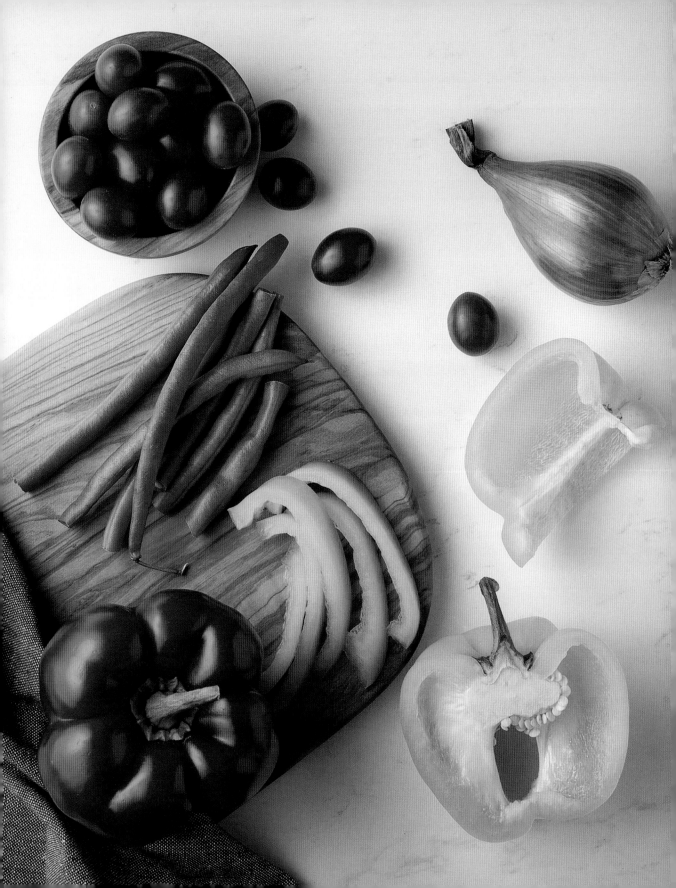

CHAPTER 1

What Is Insulin Resistance?

Metabolic conditions, such as insulin resistance, tend to travel in packs. This means that if you have one metabolic condition, you may already have another, or you may be more likely to develop another one in the future. There are many reasons why a person might develop these conditions, including both genetic and lifestyle factors. Plus, the connection between body weight and insulin resistance is complicated and surrounded by stigma. To understand this connection fully, it's important to understand both the causes and symptoms of insulin resistance. The good news is that there are many effective strategies for improving insulin resistance and other metabolic conditions.

How Do I Know If I Am Insulin Resistant?

A recent analysis of National Health and Nutrition Examination Survey (NHANES) data estimated that about 40 percent of the U.S. adult population between the ages of eighteen and forty-four are insulin resistant. Astonishingly, many people with insulin resistance are unaware that they even have the condition. Similarly, according to the 2024 Centers for Disease Control and Prevention (CDC) National Diabetes Statistics Report, "8.7 million adults aged 18 years or older who met laboratory criteria for diabetes were not aware of, or did not report having, diabetes." This means that there is a very good chance that you or someone you know either has this condition or has a high risk of developing it. Determining whether you have insulin resistance involves a combination of things: assessing your personal risk factors, observing your symptoms, and evaluating your medical laboratory tests.

Things that put you at a higher risk of insulin resistance include a family history of type 2 diabetes, a sedentary lifestyle, obesity (particularly excess fat around the abdomen), high blood pressure, and high cholesterol or high blood triglycerides. Symptoms of insulin resistance are commonly "silent" (that is, you may not always be aware of them), and include high fasting blood glucose, weight gain, and fat storage in the abdomen. In fact, most people who have insulin resistance are asymptomatic until their condition reaches the severity level of type 2 diabetes or prediabetes. To track your overall health and maintain a healthy lifestyle, it's important to visit your primary care physician annually. You might not be able to feel insulin resistance, but that doesn't mean you don't have it.

INSULIN TESTS

If you suspect you may have insulin resistance, consider asking your primary care physician for one of the following tests.

- **A1c Test:** This test, the diagnostic test for diabetes, reflects your average blood glucose level over a period of three months. This average can increase after insulin resistance has been present for an extended period of time.

- **Fasting Blood Glucose Test:** This test measures your blood glucose (blood sugar) after you have fasted for more than eight hours or overnight, and it indicates how well your body is regulating blood glucose. A rise in this lab value is often the first indicator that you are insulin resistant.

What Is Insulin Resistance?

Let's start with the basics. First of all, what is insulin and what is its function in the body? Insulin is a hormone that is produced in the pancreas and released into the bloodstream. Its main function is regulating blood glucose, but it also plays a large role in fat storage and appetite.

After you eat, your digestive system breaks down the carbohydrates in food into glucose molecules, which enter the bloodstream. The pancreas then releases insulin to help your muscles and organs absorb the glucose and use it for energy. When this process works correctly, blood glucose (blood sugar) levels remain stable. Individuals with insulin resistance, however, will experience bigger rises and falls in blood sugar.

Imagine that each cell in your body has a locked door that only opens to allow entry to important substances. Each substance needs a specific key to unlock the door so that it can move inside. In this instance, glucose is the important substance: It needs access to the cell to provide it with energy. The key that unlocks the cell door for glucose is the hormone insulin.

So far, so good. But insulin resistance occurs when your body's cells no longer respond efficiently to that "key," or hormone. Why? Most of the cells have changed their locks, so glucose can't use the insulin key to get in.

When this happens, glucose builds up in the blood, which leads to higher blood glucose levels. In response, your pancreas increases insulin production, which causes you to have both high glucose and high insulin levels in the blood.

This brings us to another of insulin's important functions: triggering fat storage. The body then responds to this scenario of higher-than-ideal blood glucose and insulin levels by storing the glucose as fat. This is one reason that insulin resistance causes weight gain, specifically around the abdomen.

WHAT IS METABOLIC SYNDROME AND HOW DOES IT RELATE TO INSULIN RESISTANCE?

Most of the people I work with through the Drop Diabetes Program also face additional metabolic conditions, such as high cholesterol, high blood pressure, polycystic ovary syndrome (PCOS), chronic kidney disease, and nonalcoholic fatty liver disease. Many, but not all, are overweight or obese.

Unfortunately, a combination of conditions like these is not unusual because metabolic conditions like company. The presence of three or more of these metabolic conditions is often referred to in the medical community as "metabolic syndrome." It increases your risk of diabetes, stroke, and heart disease and is strongly linked to insulin resistance, a sedentary lifestyle, and obesity (specifically excess fat around the abdomen).

Having insulin resistance on its own does not mean that you have metabolic syndrome, but it does mean that your risk of developing other metabolic conditions in the future is high. Making lifestyle changes is the best way to prevent this. People who make positive changes to their diets and activity levels and who manage stress effectively can prevent or significantly delay the progression of chronic conditions, most commonly high blood pressure and type 2 diabetes.

KEY TERMS

Below are definitions for a few of the terms I use in this chapter and throughout this book.

- **Blood glucose spike:** There is no medical definition of a blood glucose, or blood sugar, spike, but this term is commonly used to refer to a significant increase in blood glucose.

- **Glucose:** A molecule of sugar, it's the body's main source of energy. Glucose is found in carbohydrates in food, and it is carried in the bloodstream to be used by cells for energy. It is also stored in the liver as glycogen.

- **Glucose tolerance:** The body's ability to manage glucose levels in the blood. Impaired glucose tolerance indicates early signs of insulin resistance. It's sometimes referred to as "carb tolerance."

- **Glycemic index:** The scale that indicates the effect a specific food will have on blood sugar. The higher the glycemic index of a food, the more likely it is to raise blood sugar.

- **Hyperinsulinemia:** A condition in which the pancreas produces too much insulin in order to compensate for insulin resistance. High insulin levels can contribute to weight gain and fat storage.

- **Insulin resistance:** A condition in which the body's cells become less responsive to insulin, requiring the pancreas to produce more insulin to allow glucose to enter the cells. This can lead to elevated blood glucose levels.

- **Insulin sensitivity:** This refers to how effectively the body's cells respond to insulin. High insulin sensitivity means that the body efficiently responds to insulin and that carb tolerance is high. Low insulin sensitivity means that the body does not respond efficiently to insulin and carb tolerance is likely to be low.

- **Metabolic syndrome:** A cluster of conditions—including insulin resistance, high blood pressure, elevated cholesterol, and excess abdominal fat—that increases the risk of type 2 diabetes and heart disease.

- **Pancreas:** An organ that produces insulin and other digestive enzymes. The pancreas responds to rising blood sugar levels by releasing insulin to help lower them.

- **Prediabetes:** A condition in which blood glucose levels are higher than normal but not high enough to be classified as type 2 diabetes. It is diagnosed by an A1c result of between 5.7 and 6.4 percent. It's an early warning sign that the body is not using insulin effectively, often due to insulin resistance. Without intervention, such as lifestyle changes, prediabetes can progress into type 2 diabetes. A prediabetes diagnosis is a critical window for reversing or preventing the onset of full diabetes.

- **Type 2 diabetes:** A chronic condition in which the body becomes resistant to insulin, leading to high blood sugar levels and potentially serious health complications. Type 2 diabetes is diagnosed by an A1c result of 6.5 percent or higher.

What Causes Insulin Resistance?

The exact cause of insulin resistance is not fully understood by the medical community, though several things have been proven to contribute to it. These include:

Genetics: A family history of related conditions can affect your predisposition to insulin resistance and developing diabetes or being overweight. That said, while genetics may put you at a higher risk of certain conditions, it doesn't mean that you're definitely going to develop them. While it is common knowledge that genes are passed down to us by our parents, many of us forget that lifestyle habits are also passed down from generation to generation. You might not be able to alter your genes, but you can change your habits.

Hormonal imbalances: Cushing's syndrome, PCOS, Hashimoto's disease, and other hormonal conditions can affect insulin sensitivity, which means they can lead to other metabolic disorders such as insulin resistance.

Poor stress management: Stress triggers your adrenal glands to release a hormone called cortisol into the bloodstream. Cortisol causes your liver to release stored glucose, which leads to increased blood glucose. The pancreas is then triggered to release insulin in response, resulting in a vicious cycle. Chronic stress causes this trifecta of high cortisol, glucose, and insulin to remain in the blood for long periods of time and can result in insulin resistance as well as weight gain. Ever wonder why you find it difficult to lose weight, despite your best efforts? Chronic stress may play a role.

Inactivity: Physical activity builds muscle and trains those muscle cells to absorb glucose and use insulin efficiently, thus improving insulin sensitivity. A long-term lack of physical activity can have the opposite effect, causing your cells to use insulin inefficiently. That's why a sedentary lifestyle can contribute to weight gain and insulin resistance, among other health risks.

Diet: A diet that frequently includes highly processed foods and foods high in carbohydrates and saturated fats has been linked to insulin resistance. Here's why: Your body digests processed, high-carb foods very quickly, causing blood glucose levels to spike. This puts additional stress on the pancreas to produce and release an unusually high amount of insulin. Eventually, the pancreas gets tired of putting in overtime and may reduce its insulin output, and the cells in the body become resistant to the insulin that it does produce.

Excess body fat: Medical scientists believe that obesity, especially excess fat around the abdomen and the organs (visceral fat), is a primary cause of insulin resistance. This hypothesis needs further research, due to the convoluted data available on whether insulin resistance causes weight gain or weight gain causes insulin resistance, a "which came first: the chicken or the egg?" sort of dilemma. Since the subject of weight and insulin resistance is complex and often misunderstood, let's take a moment to clarify the connection between them.

WEIGHT AND INSULIN RESISTANCE

First, let's be clear: Obesity can cause insulin resistance because it places the body in a state in which it struggles to produce and use insulin effectively. The accumulation of excess body fat around the abdomen, muscles, and organs, particularly the liver, interferes with the way your body signals the release and use of insulin. This makes it harder for your cells to absorb glucose from the blood. Fat cells also release inflammatory markers, which activate a stress response that blocks insulin from reaching its receptors.

However, it's important to note that this works in the other direction as well: Insulin resistance can cause weight gain because of the role insulin plays in storing nutrients in the body. When cells become insulin resistant and blood insulin levels rise, fat storage is triggered. Since the level of insulin in the blood remains high for long periods of time, the body receives constant messaging to store, rather than burn, fat. Additionally, the presence of insulin resistance is often disruptive to the hormone leptin, which signals fullness, and this can cause overeating.

While it is true that visceral fat can increase hormones that lead to insulin resistance, it would be misleading to assume that excess fat is the only thing that *causes* the insulin resistance. Understanding this dichotomy is essential to understanding why a simple calorie-restricted weight loss approach alone will not lower insulin resistance and weight. This is not to say that weight loss is a bad goal to have, but the truth is that common weight loss efforts do not consider the bigger picture of overall metabolic health. The big takeaway here is that we cannot simply blame insulin resistance on excess weight and focus strictly on weight loss because, in most cases, this does not solve the problem of insulin resistance.

THE STIGMA SURROUNDING INSULIN RESISTANCE AND DIABETES

We need to pause here to address the stigma around insulin resistance, weight, and type 2 diabetes. It's a common misconception that a poor diet is the main cause of type 2 diabetes. People with type 2 diabetes are labelled as terribly inactive or even lazy. But, as I mentioned earlier, the truth is that there are a lot of reasons why insulin resistance might crop up, including genetics, stress, and hormonal conditions, which are nobody's fault.

Another common misconception is that people with insulin resistance should stop eating carbohydrates and are generally limited in what they can eat. While it is true that most people with insulin resistance do need to make dietary modifications, a drastic approach is not the answer.

The Long-Term Effects of Insulin Resistance

If it isn't addressed, insulin resistance can escalate and cause a variety of health complications. The most common of these is type 2 diabetes, due to higher-than-normal blood glucose levels having been present for an extended period of time. However, chronically high blood glucose levels caused by insulin resistance can lead to a host of other issues, such as kidney damage, vision impairment, and nerve damage (neuropathy).

Insulin resistance is also linked to increased triglycerides and LDL cholesterol levels, leading to a higher risk of heart disease, heart attack, and stroke. If a person with insulin resistance has visceral fat, they are likely to develop non-alcoholic fatty liver disease (NAFLD), which can progress into liver failure. Metabolic syndrome, which can include the above conditions, is common in people with insulin resistance. In women, insulin resistance can contribute to the onset of polycystic ovarian syndrome (PCOS), a hormonal disorder that affects fertility, causes irregular menstrual cycles, and increases the risk of diabetes.

Can Insulin Resistance Be Reversed?

Current medical research indicates that, with lifestyle modifications, insulin resistance can be put into remission. That's "remission," not "reversal." Using the term "reversed" in conjunction with the treatment of insulin resistance is misleading. The term "remission" is much more accurate in describing the outlook that the research suggests an individual can achieve.

In terms of insulin resistance, "remission" means that a person has reached a stage where their blood glucose and insulin levels are well controlled. This does not mean that their insulin resistance is permanently gone; it means that the lifestyle patterns they are currently maintaining are managing their condition well.

Read the previous paragraph again. The most important keyword there is "maintaining." If you are hoping to reach remission, it is of the utmost importance that you are making changes you can maintain for the rest of your life. This is where fad dieting has done people a great disservice: It has hindered their efforts to improve their metabolic health, causing extreme fluctuations in eating patterns, weight, metabolic rate, and hormonal balance. Each decade has had its stack of fad diets, but time and again the research shows that, for most of the population (aside from those with major health conditions or allergies), a balanced eating pattern filled with fruits, vegetables, lean proteins, and whole grains is the best approach.

Actionable Steps to Improve Insulin Resistance

Now let's talk about the lifestyle modifications you can make to reach remission. As you read on, it's important to remember that everyone has unique needs, lifestyle factors, and health goals. There is no one-size-fits-all approach to nutrition (regardless of the presence or absence of any particular health condition). This is why it's essential to get support in finding an eating pattern and lifestyle that is sustainable for you personally, based on some key principles.

Before we discuss those principles, it's helpful to consider how diet culture may have affected your own diet and the way you've approached food throughout your life. For many people, restrictive diets have been a part of life for years. It might surprise you to learn that restrictive dieting is associated with worsening health conditions, such as metabolic slowdown, hormonal imbalances, nutrient deficiencies, muscle loss, and weight gain. To reach remission and prevent metabolic conditions, we want to focus on an eating pattern that's nutritious overall rather than narrowing our vision and following a specific diet program or restricting specific nutrients, such as carbohydrates.

The following four categories of lifestyle changes will not only help improve insulin resistance, but also promote weight loss, boost metabolic health, and even enhance mobility. Most individuals thrive when they start out slowly, introducing one change, or a few small changes, at a time. Small changes truly do lead to big results. Meet yourself where you are today, because Rome wasn't built in a day (and neither were your biceps). Let's take action.

INCORPORATE REGULAR PHYSICAL ACTIVITY INTO YOUR DAY

A sedentary lifestyle increases your risk for metabolic conditions, including insulin resistance.

Physical activity builds muscle and trains that muscle to use insulin more efficiently to better absorb glucose from the blood. A long-term lack of physical activity can have the opposite effect, causing insulin resistance. Additionally, a sedentary lifestyle is associated with weight gain, which can also contribute to insulin resistance.

Remember the lock and key analogy we used to visualize how insulin functions in admitting glucose into our cells? Insulin resistance happens when your cells change the locks. But exercise, such as moderate intensity walking or strength training, can "unlock" your cells from the inside. Muscle activity triggers GLUT4 transporters (a protein in muscle cells that helps move glucose into the cell) to move to the cell surface, where they unlock the cell's "doors" from the inside. This is one of the many benefits of exercise, but it is especially important for people with insulin resistance.

Aerobic activities like walking, running, swimming, biking, and dancing are great ways to maintain or improve your cardiovascular and metabolic health. These forms of exercise increase your metabolic rate—how quickly you burn energy—and help your cells use insulin more efficiently.

The basic guideline for aerobic activity is 150 minutes per week, or 30 minutes, five days per week. Consistency is crucial here: Doing 30 minutes of aerobic exercise most days of the week instead of, say, 75 minutes twice weekly, will give you the most cardiovascular and metabolic benefits.

While it's important to prioritize aerobic activity, the most beneficial form of exercise for reducing insulin resistance is strength training, which builds muscle. This can include weight lifting, body-weight movements, or movements that use resistance bands or other exercise equipment to support muscle building. Increased muscle mass means you have more muscle to use up the glucose in your bloodstream. It also improves insulin sensitivity by training your muscles to use insulin more efficiently.

Adding a strength-training activity to your exercise routine two or three times per week is a great starting place. Remember not to try to do too much too fast. Meet yourself where you are: If you are a beginner, start with just 5 to 10 minutes of your chosen activity. If you are more advanced, try 30 minutes.

High-intensity interval training (HIIT) exercise incorporates both strengthening and cardio movements and can accommodate both aerobic and muscle-building exercises. Try doing this in lieu of your cardiovascular workout one to two times per week.

Exercise is important, but so is recovery. Choose activities like gentle yoga, stretching, or walking at a leisurely pace on your recovery days. Ultimately, getting 30 minutes of physical activity daily will improve insulin sensitivity immensely.

PRIORITIZE SLEEP

Your body heals and regulates hormones while you sleep. For this reason, a lack of adequate sleep, or poor-quality sleep, will affect the body's insulin sensitivity. Poor sleep is associated with higher blood glucose numbers in the morning, which is commonly referred to as the "dawn phenomenon." This is a natural rise in blood glucose levels in the early morning due to increased production of hormones like cortisol and adrenaline, which trigger the liver to release glucose for quick energy when you wake up in a state of

fasting. In the presence of insulin resistance, this mechanism is mis-regulated, and blood glucose can rise to a less-than-ideal level. This explains why high fasting blood glucose is an indicator of insulin resistance.

So, if you get less than seven hours of sleep per night, consider how you spend your time and see if you can change your schedule to ensure that you get between seven and nine hours of sleep per night.

If you have trouble sleeping, consider improving your bedtime routine. Avoid screen time and do an activity that helps you physically and mentally wind down, like reading, taking a bath, or stretching. If you feel anxious or tense at bedtime, try journaling, meditating, or writing a quick to-do list for the following day to avoid thinking about all the things you need to do.

If you have significant or chronic trouble sleeping, setting an action plan for improving sleep quality or hours of sleep is important. Consult a doctor if your sleep quality doesn't improve with habit changes, as it may be a sign of vitamin D deficiency or other issues.

FOCUS ON STRESS MANAGEMENT

Chronic stress plays a large role in developing and accelerating insulin resistance. When you experience stress, whether physical or emotional, cortisol and adrenaline enter the bloodstream to put your body into fight-or-flight mode. This causes blood glucose and then insulin to rise, and so on, and you're back in the same cycle described on page 15.

Some stress in life is inevitable, yes, but chronic stress can lead to weight gain and insulin resistance regardless of other lifestyle factors. Stress also makes us more likely to make negative lifestyle choices, such as overeating, being inactive, and sleeping poorly. This is why stress can create a waterfall effect on your health, and that means managing it well is vital. Write out a list of your regular stressors. Are any of these avoidable? Is there anything that is no longer serving you from which you can take a step back? Is there someone you can delegate to or who can help you with your unique stressors?

We live in a hectic world where we are always pressured to do more. Many of us have high-stress work environments, busy home lives, or both. The following techniques are just some of the ways that you can reduce or manage your stress.

Connect with others: Interaction with friends and loved ones brings joy, support, and a sense of connection.

Practice meditation or deep breathing: Mindfulness is a great practice for clearing your thoughts and improving focus.

Practice gratitude: Having a regular gratitude practice has been shown to alleviate stress and improve mood in individuals suffering from stress and conditions such as anxiety and depression.

Try yoga: The mind-body connection in yoga practice promotes calm and a sense of peace, reducing stress in the process. Even a few minutes can release the tension that you may be holding in your muscles. It's also great for your spine, and certain types of higher-intensity yoga promote muscle building, supporting overall health.

Go for a walk: Walking for 10 to 15 minutes when you feel stressed can reduce your blood glucose levels and help regulate hormones.

Limit your caffeine intake: Excessive caffeine intake has been linked to higher anxiety and stress levels. The basic guideline for caffeine consumption is less than 400 milligrams per day, or about 16 ounces (240 ml) of coffee.

Limit your exposure to social media and news: "Doomscrolling" on social media or watching negative news stories can worsen mood, increase stress, and even decrease focus and attention span. Be mindful of the platforms from which you get your information and entertainment: Are they helping or harming you?

Engage with a hobby that brings you joy: Read a book for fun, play a game, do something outdoors, create art, cook, garden, or simply take time to fully relax your mind.

Take a few minutes to reflect on what helps you release stress and feel at peace. How can you regularly incorporate even one of these strategies into your life? After reflection, create an action plan (I'll discuss this technique fully in chapter 2).

EAT A BALANCED, NUTRIENT-DENSE DIET

What does a balanced, healthy eating pattern look like?

A balanced eating pattern includes a variety of nutrient-dense foods, including carbohydrates in the form of whole grains and fruit, lean proteins, vegetables, nuts, and legumes. Choosing minimally processed foods—that is, foods that haven't been stripped of their natural fiber, vitamins, or minerals and have very little added sugar or saturated fat—is always best.

You'll also want to avoid fad diets. When you investigate them, you'll notice that most fad diets have a restrictive factor. They may be, say, calorie-restricted, carb-restricted, or fat-restricted. However, restricting a specific macronutrient or food group removes the balance that the human body needs. For that reason, you will notice that there is no diet specific emphasis in this cookbook. There are ways to enjoy eating to reduce insulin resistance without being on a regimented or restrictive diet.

The Elements of an Insulin-Friendly Diet

The goal of an insulin-friendly eating pattern is to improve carb tolerance, reduce insulin resistance, and prevent additional metabolic conditions from arising. This eating pattern emphasizes mostly whole foods and limits (but does not completely cut out) highly processed foods. It does not over-restrict carbohydrates, instead focusing on increasing carb tolerance. It is comprised of healthy carbohydrates, lean proteins (both animal- and plant-based), nonstarchy vegetables, and foods that are rich in omega-3 fatty acids. It emphasizes high-fiber foods and reasonably limits foods that are high in saturated fat, sodium, refined carbohydrates, and added sugar.

An insulin-friendly eating pattern includes foods containing:

Healthy carbohydrates. Wholesome carbohydrate foods also contain fiber and essential micronutrients that are important for overall metabolic health. These include fruits; starchy vegetables such as potatoes, peas and squash; whole grains; legumes; and dairy products. It's not just about the grams of carbohydrate per serving, it's also about the composition of that food and how you consume it. Foods high in carbohydrates can be healthy.

Lean proteins. Getting 30 grams of protein per meal is a great goal for improving insulin resistance. Choose options that are minimally processed and low in saturated fats. Both animal and plant sources of protein are acceptable, such as chicken, fish, tofu, and beans.

Nonstarchy vegetables. Vegetables such as leafy greens, broccoli, cauliflower, carrots, and tomatoes are high in fiber, vitamins, and minerals. Try to eat at least 3 cups of vegetables daily, and more is even better.

Omega-3 fatty acids. Inflammation in the body contributes to insulin resistance. Foods rich in omega-3 fatty acids, such as fatty fish, avocadoes, and nuts, help to reduce inflammation.

Fiber. Fiber is an important nutrient for regulating digestion, improving gut health, maintaining fullness, stabilizing blood sugar, and lowering cholesterol levels. Fiber-rich foods include beans, lentils, nuts, seeds, vegetables, and whole grains.

A healthy eating pattern reasonably limits foods containing:

Saturated fat. Excess saturated fat can cause inflammation, impaired liver function, cardiovascular conditions, and excess weight gain. A diet high in saturated fat has been shown to worsen insulin resistance.

Sodium. Consuming too much sodium is easy to do, thanks to the prevalence of processed foods and convenience items, as well as restaurant culture. If you have insulin resistance, limiting this nutrient is important due to your increased risk of cardiovascular conditions.

Refined carbohydrates. Foods that contain refined carbohydrates are why carbs get a bad rep. During processing, refined carbs are stripped of most of their natural fiber, vitamins, and minerals. They raise blood sugar quickly and are not nutritious. Refined carbohydrates are commonly found in white breads, baked goods, candies, and soda.

Added sugar. When sugar occurs naturally in foods, it occurs in moderate amounts. But when manufacturers add sugar to foods, they typically add it in excess. Consuming excess added sugar can increase insulin resistance, so you should watch out for it. The recommended daily limit on added sugar is 25 grams. Remember that this does not include sugars naturally occurring in foods such as fruit and milk.

An important factor in any successful eating pattern is sustainability. While certain foods are not helpful in reducing insulin resistance, they are important for food satisfaction, pleasure, and enjoyment. Let's call these "fun foods" and consider ways to make them fit into your eating pattern. For example, birthday cake may not be a wholesome food, but it is a tradition that you don't need to miss out on for the rest of your life. Similarly, family pizza night may be an important bonding experience for you and your kids. Whatever your fun foods are, don't cut them out; enjoy them in moderation instead. Realistically, you'll want to enjoy an ice cream cone at some point in the future. An insulin-friendly eating pattern isn't about perfection: It's about making mostly wholesome choices and enjoying fun foods in a sustainable way.

TYPES OF CARBOHYDRATES

Let's talk about carbohydrates. You've probably heard a lot of mixed messages about them. Are they good, bad, or somewhere in between? Well, here's the truth: Not all carbs are created equal, and the key to keeping your blood sugar steady is choosing the right ones.

A carbohydrate is one of the three macronutrients that provide energy to the body, along with protein and fat. Carbs are the only nutrient that directly raises blood sugar, which is why they are often made out to be enemies of people with insulin resistance or type 2 diabetes. But once you understand the types of carbohydrates, you'll see their importance and the positive impact they have on your health.

Carbs can be broken down into three categories:

Simple carbohydrates. Also known as sugars, simple carbs are short chains of glucose that are digested quickly. They are found in fruits, milk, honey, maple syrup, and, of course, white sugar.

Complex carbohydrates. Complex carbs, or starches, are longer chains of glucose that your body breaks down more slowly. They are found in grains, starchy vegetables, beans, and legumes.

Fiber. Fiber has a different function than starch and sugar. It is found in both simple carbs (fruits) and complex carbs (starchy vegetables, grains, beans and legumes). Fiber is also found in foods that don't contain a significant amount of carbohydrates, such as nuts, seeds, and nonstarchy vegetables. Aim to consume 30 grams of fiber per day, and try to get your fiber from food sources instead of supplements.

The Right Way to Eat Carbohydrates

Here's how to consume carbs to improve your insulin resistance:

- Choose carbs that contain at least 3 to 5 grams of fiber per serving.

- Strive for whole, unprocessed or lightly processed foods. For example, choose whole fruit over fruit juice, whole-grain bread over white bread, and whole grain or chickpea pasta over white pasta.

- Pair fiber-rich carbs with a protein and a vegetable for a full meal. If snacking, simply pair them with a protein-rich food.

- Limit refined grains. Choose whole grains such as quinoa, wild rice, whole-grain bread or pasta. While you don't have to completely cut out refined pasta and bread, you should limit your intake of them.

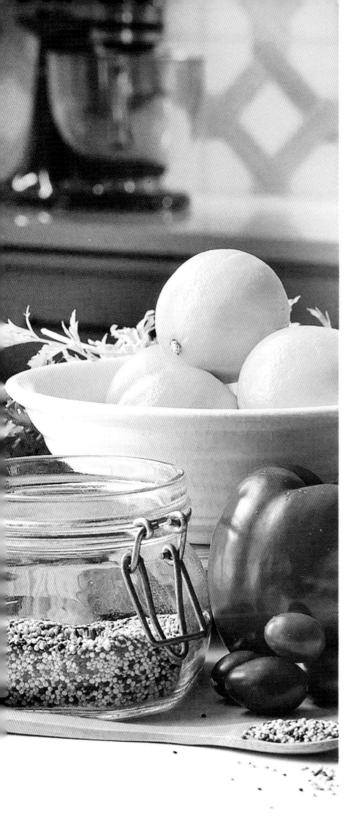

Remember, it's not about cutting out carbs—it's about choosing the right ones and eating them alongside additional protein, fiber, and fat. With a few simple swaps and mindful combinations, you can enjoy your favorite foods while reducing insulin resistance.

HOW THIS BOOK ALIGNS WITH THESE PRINCIPLES

The recipes in this book emphasize these insulin-friendly nutrition principles and balanced food-pairing techniques. Each meal is correctly balanced and contains ingredients that are high in fiber, protein, and omega-3 fatty acids. You'll also find that most of the ingredients are minimally processed.

Where one or two ingredients are high in saturated fat, such as the bacon in my Insulin-Friendly Carbonara (page 88) and the beef in my Slow-Cooker Braised Roast with Root Vegetables (page 98), the recipes' cooking methods will reduce the fat while maintaining flavor. Sodium is kept to a minimum (while maintaining the integrity of the recipe). The same goes for added sugar; this appears only in the form of honey, which has a lower glycemic index than refined sugar.

Now that you understand what insulin resistance is and how to put it into remission, let's talk about implementing the strategies discussed so far. Understanding how to improve your health is one piece of the puzzle, but it can only create a health transformation if you turn it into an action plan to help you create meaningful lifestyle changes.

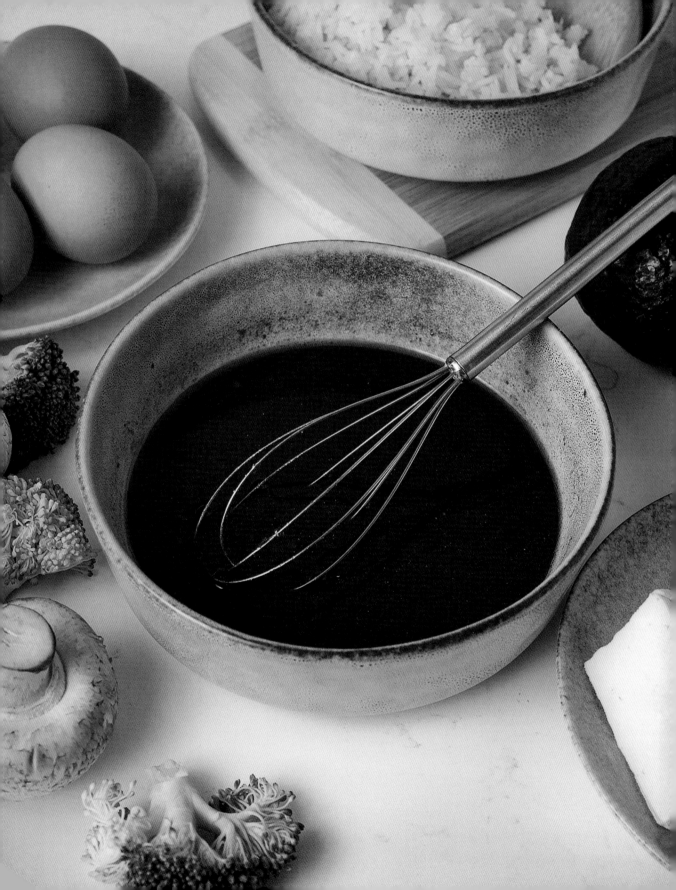

CHAPTER 2

Implementing Your Insulin-Resistance Action Plan

Now that you have a basic understanding of what insulin resistance is, I'm going to introduce you to meal planning, show you how to set up your own insulin-friendly kitchen, and give you action plans to help you reach your health goals. You'll see that a healthy, insulin-friendly eating pattern isn't about bland recipes full of obscure and expensive ingredients. It's based on familiar foods, reasonable portions, and plenty of flavor.

By now, you know the basic principles of an insulin-friendly eating pattern. You're probably already committed to making positive changes to your diet, and you may already have an idea of what those changes will look like. The next step is setting up an action plan to implement what you've learned into your day-to-day routine.

Remember, you don't have to be perfect, and you don't have to do everything at once. Build your meal plan by adding one or two new recipes each week, and watch your collection of favorites grow. Make notes on your favorite recipes and ingredient swaps. Each recipe is a complete, balanced meal or snack with notes that show you how to adapt it if you have food allergies or specific diet preferences, so you'll be able to tailor them to your own taste.

Finally, don't forget that there's no such thing as one-size-fits-all when it comes to improving your health in the long term. The key is developing a realistic approach that you can stick to and enjoy.

Stocking Your Insulin-Friendly Kitchen

Most people think that they need to clean out the pantry when they're diagnosed with a health condition like insulin resistance, but by now you've learned that you don't need to cut any foods out altogether (it's okay to have treats like ice cream in the freezer). To avoid over-restriction and the subsequent falling off the wagon, don't get into the all-or-nothing mindset of keeping the number of "fun foods" in your home at absolute zero. If, say, 80 to 90 percent of the foods in your house are wholesome (that is, they consist of high-fiber foods, lean proteins, healthy fats, fruits, veggies), you're set up for success.

Having a supply of these staple foods on hand means you'll have many of the ingredients for the recipes in this book. Stocking these ingredients also comes in handy when life gets in the way, your meal plan falls through, and you need to pull something together quickly. While it's true that making food from scratch is best, some shortcuts are worthwhile, such as jars of minced garlic, bottles of lemon and lime juice, grated Parmesan cheese, canned beans, and canned chicken. The foods in the following lists are a great starting point, but don't feel as if you have to invest in everything. Take what works for you and leave the rest. These lists are here for your reference. Feel free to add notes so you can keep track of your own favorite staple foods.

In the refrigerator:

- "Ready to eat" vegetables you can grab on the go, such as carrots, celery, bell peppers, cherry tomatoes, and so on
- Fruits: Choose two of your favorites each week, and vary them based on seasonal availability

- Condiments and common ingredients
  - Minced garlic (preserved in oil)
  - Salsa
  - Almond milk
  - Grated Parmesan cheese (the pre-grated kind is fine)
  - Lemon and lime juice
- Proteins
  - 2% low-fat milk
  - Nonfat plain Greek yogurt
  - Feta cheese
  - Cheese sticks or cheese cubes
  - Shredded mozzarella
  - Cottage cheese
  - Low-fat ricotta cheese
  - Eggs
  - Rotisserie chicken
  - Chicken apple sausage
  - Firm or extra firm tofu

In the freezer:

- Frozen boneless skinless chicken, beef, pork, turkey, fish
- Frozen vegetables (broccoli, peas, kale, spinach, cauliflower rice, and so on)
- Frozen berries (blueberries, strawberries, blackberries, and so on)

In the pantry:

- Condiments and common ingredients
  - Cooking spray (olive or avocado oil)
  - Olive oil
  - Avocado oil
  - Toasted sesame oil
  - Low-sodium soy sauce
  - Coconut aminos
  - Balsamic vinegar
  - Apple cider vinegar
  - Red wine vinegar
  - A variety of dried herbs and spices
- Vegetables
  - Onions
  - Potatoes
  - Sweet potatoes
  - Tomatoes

WHAT IS A SUGAR ALTERNATIVE BAKING BLEND?

Traditional non-caloric sweeteners are 200 to 300 times sweeter than sugar, making them challenging to use in baking because they lack the bulk and structural properties of sugar. Sugar alternative baking blends solve this problem by incorporating bulking agents like erythritol, which mimic sugar's texture and volume. This allows for a seamless 1 to 1 substitution, making these blends a practical choice for recipes that require sugar's unique functionality in baking.

- Grains
  - Sourdough or whole-grain bread
  - 8-inch (20 cm) Ole Xtreme high fiber tortillas
  - 5-inch (13 cm) corn tortillas
  - Oats (old-fashioned)
  - Quinoa, farro, wild rice, and so on
  - Jasmine or basmati rice
  - Whole-grain pasta
  - Chickpea or lentil pasta
  - Microwaveable quinoa cups (for use in a pinch)
- Nuts and seeds
  - Cashews, walnuts, pecans, almonds, and so on
  - Chia, flax, hemp, sunflower seeds, and so on
- Proteins
  - Canned chicken breast
  - Flavored tuna packs
  - Canned beans (chickpeas, black beans, cannellini beans, and so on)
  - Natural sugar-free peanut butter
- Baking staples
  - White and brown sugar alternative baking blends (such as Swerve or Truvia)
  - Your favorite alternative sweetener (such as sugar-free maple-flavored syrup or monk fruit)
  - Sugar-free chocolate chips (such as Lily's brand)
  - Honey
- Snacks and supplements
  - Popcorn kernels (for popping at home)
  - Crispy chickpeas, store-bought or homemade
  - Whole-grain or seed crackers
  - Vanilla protein powder

RECOMMENDED KITCHEN TOOLS

Stocking your kitchen isn't just about food. Here's a list of kitchen tools that you'll need as you prepare the recipes in this book.

- Sheet pans: half (18 by 13 inches / 45 by 33 cm) and quarter (9½ by 13 inches / 24 by 33 cm)
- Small, medium, and large pots and skillets
- 9 by 13-inch (23 by 33 cm) baking dish
- Small, medium, and large metal mixing bowls
- Cutting boards
- Food processor
- Blender
- Hand mixer
- Measuring cups and spoons
- Parchment paper
- Utensils:
  - Whisk
  - Rubber or silicone spatula
  - Wooden spoons
  - Standard metal or silicone spatula
  - Ladle
  - Tongs
  - Chef's knife
  - Paring knife

SIX KITCHEN HACKS THAT MAKE LIFE EASIER

Use vinegar after you cook fish or broccoli to keep the kitchen smelling fresh. Place a small bowl of white vinegar on the counter overnight to absorb any leftover odors.

Keep pre-cut produce fresh. Avocados and apples will brown when cut and left uncovered. To keep them fresh, place them in the refrigerator in an airtight container with a few drops of lemon juice. The acid in the lemon juice will slow the chemical reaction of browning, keeping them fresh for longer.

Avoid tears when cutting onions. Acid released from the onion during cutting darts to the nearest water source, which is usually your eyes. Placing a wet cloth or paper towel next to your onion while you're cutting it will absorb the acid and make it a tear-free experience.

Veggie choppers make your life easier. The recipes in this book don't require specialized equipment, but I do recommend investing in a veggie chopper to save time and spare your sanity when you're making any recipe that requires slicing and dicing. These can be found affordably online or at most department stores.

Ripen an avocado at home. Place the avocado in a paper bag with a banana. As the banana ripens, it produces ethylene, which speeds up the ripening process so you won't have to wait forever to use your avocado.

Measure sticky ingredients (like peanut butter) without the mess by lightly spraying your measuring cup with cooking spray. Use a rubber spatula to scoop out the measured ingredient, and you'll have a much easier time cleaning up.

Meal Planning

Hungry people make rash decisions. When we get hungry, we have less patience for decision-making, so we often choose convenience foods or go out to eat to avoid putting thought into it. If you're already confused about what to eat due to a metabolic condition such as insulin resistance, you're even more likely to make less-than-ideal choices. Meal planning ensures that you have plenty of healthy foods on hand so that you're never caught short.

That said, when it comes to making healthy lifestyle changes, practice makes perfect. You don't need to change everything about your eating pattern all at once, and your meal plans don't have to be perfect, either. Meal planning should be simple and fun and shouldn't take hours of your time. By following my meal planning strategy, you'll be able to quickly put together a week of meals that work both for your body and your busy schedule.

Still, sometimes plans fall apart (even when you're a diabetes dietitian), which is why this section also includes fail-safes to see you through even the busiest days.

MEGAN'S FAVORITE MEAL PLANNING TOOL

It's a good idea to have a planner dedicated to meals: Try putting it on your refrigerator or in an easily accessible drawer. Your planner can take the form of a dry erase board, a calendar, a big sticky note, or any other medium that suits you. I also recommend keeping your grocery list right next to it.

I have a weekly meal planner dry-erase board with a notes section that I found online. This way, my whole family can see what meals are planned for the week and what's available for breakfast and snacks. I also add scheduling notes, such as "tennis practice" or "yoga, 6:30 to 7:30 pm" to the planner, so that we're all on the same page and can prep meals accordingly.

MEGAN'S 15-MINUTE MEAL-PLANNING STRATEGY

This is the meal-planning strategy that I have used for years, and I'm excited to share it with you. While it's true that different things work for different people, my six-step strategy is a great starting point. Mold it into a plan that works for you, and start small to avoid feeling over-whelmed. Try making one or two small changes per week (or per month), instead of trying to change everything at once. This process may take you a little more than 15 minutes at first, but the more often you do it, the faster it'll become.

Here's an overview of the process:

- **Step 1:** Map out your week (time: 1 to 2 minutes)

- **Step 2:** Select five dinner recipes (time: 4 to 5 minutes)

- **Step 3:** Add in two to three breakfast recipes, two to three lunch recipes, and two to three snack recipes (time: 4 to 5 minutes)

- **Step 4:** Make your shopping list (time: 4 to 5 minutes)

- **Step 5:** Shop at the same time every week

- **Step 6:** Do your meal prep

Step 1. Map out your week: Think about the week ahead: Do you have an especially busy evening, a day with no time at all to cook, or a business trip? You can plan for that. Plan a slow-cooker meal for busy nights, or plan to cook a double batch earlier in the week for leftovers. Or pencil in a meal that doesn't require cooking, such as many of the 5- to 15-minute lunch recipes in chapter 4.

Step 2. Select five dinner recipes: This is the easiest step of all. Turn to chapter 5 and pick five recipes that sound good to you this week. Put them on the plan. Keep it flexible, though; you don't have to commit to a specific night for each meal, unless step 1 tells you so.

SHREDDED CHICKEN

Multiple recipes in this book call for cooked and shredded chicken breasts. To prepare this, season boneless chicken breasts with salt and pepper and bake at 375°F (190°C) for 20 to 25 minutes until the internal temperature reaches 165°F (75°C). Let the chicken rest for 5 minutes, then shred with two forks or a stand mixer with a paddle attachment.

MORE KITCHEN TIPS AND SHORTCUTS

Easily and safely cut an avocado with no mess by slicing it in half lengthwise around the pit with a chef's knife. Ease the two halves apart and remove the pit carefully. If you want to slice the avocado flesh, do this while it is still inside the skin; then scoop out gently with a large spoon.

Press tofu for 10 to 30 minutes before using it in a recipe. No special equipment is required. Place two paper towels on a flat plate. Put the tofu on the plate, then top with two more paper towels and another flat plate turned upside down. Finally, place something heavy onto the top plate (such as large hardcover books) to put pressure on the tofu and squeeze out excess liquid, then use the pressed tofu as directed.

Save time by cutting large chicken breasts in half horizontally to make two thinner cutlets. This method reduces the cooking time significantly (and results in more realistic portions). Cubing chicken before cooking is also a great time saver.

Step 3. Add two to three breakfast recipes, two to three lunch recipes, and two to three snack recipes: Another easy one. Browse through chapters 3 and 6 to find breakfasts and snacks that you'd like to make this week. Some are easily prepped ahead of time for busy weekdays; others take only a few minutes to make in the morning. Repeat those breakfasts and snacks throughout the week.

Step 4. Make your shopping list: As you select your recipes for the week, add the ingredients for them to your grocery list. Make sure to check your kitchen for any ingredients that you may already have so you don't double up.

Step 5. Shop at the same time every week: Pick a day of the week that works best for you to do your grocery shopping. A routine will be your friend here. For example, I always do my meal plan on Thursday evenings, and my grocery shopping on Saturday mornings. Which day works well for you? Pick it and stick to it.

Step 6. Meal prep: You've probably seen people posting on social media about their "Meal Prep Sunday" strategy. But who has a whole afternoon to devote to cooking and packaging? Most of us would agree that that's mighty ambitious. So here's my time-saving approach to meal prep:

> **When:** I don't do all my meal prep on one particular day. Instead, I meal prep while I'm making dinner and am already being active in the kitchen. For example, while your soup is simmering or your meal is in the oven and you're not actively cooking, use that time to do meal prep for the week. Boil eggs, make an oatmeal bake (page 58), or cut vegetables.

> **What:** The simple stuff. I prep things that are uncomplicated and easy to do in advance, such as boiling eggs, cooking quinoa or farro, roasting vegetables, cutting up veggies, washing fruit, or whipping up the Prep-ahead Crustless Mini Quiches on

COOKING FOR ONE

Many recipes make multiple portions, so cooking for one can be a bit tricky, but don't let that keep you from eating well. You are worth the effort. Here are a few ways to make it easier.

Adjust ingredient quantities: For the recipe you choose, divide each ingredient quantity by two (or even three, depending on the number of servings it makes) and write in the new quantity for each ingredient. You can use this technique for any recipe in this book. If an ingredient comes out to a nonstandard quantity when adjusted (for example: ⅓ teaspoon), estimating to the best of your ability will usually work fine.

Make freezer meals: Alternatively, you can prepare full recipes and freeze the leftovers in individual glass containers. This way you'll have plenty of pre-made meals on hand for busy nights when you don't have time to cook, or for when you come home from a business trip or weekend away and have no fresh food in the kitchen.

Batch cook: Prepare two meals per week for both lunch and dinner and have the leftovers on the remaining days. This is an excellent way to enjoy leftovers without getting bored.

page 49 for breakfast all week. Essentially, if the task is low-focus and takes only a few minutes to complete, you can get it done ahead of time in this way.

Action Planning

Action planning starts with creating a list of the changes or habits that must happen to achieve a goal. Then you'll take an item from this list and break it down into specific action steps to implement it. This technique can really help you to set yourself up for successful lifestyle change. Do this 10-minute process weekly to keep yourself accountable and to keep your goals in sight.

THE ACTION PLANNING PROCESS

First, take a moment to write down your main long-term health goal. This goal should answer the question: What do I ultimately want to achieve that would make me feel as if I am moving forward in my health journey?

Next, take a moment to write down your shorter-term goals. What are one or two things that you can start doing now that will bring you closer to your main goal above? For example, if your main goal is to put insulin resistance into remission, you could work on increasing your daily physical activity and implementing a more insulin-friendly eating pattern.

Now, get even more specific. What do you need to do to implement those smaller goals? Note that an action plan is meant to continually build habits in the long term, and does not have an end date. So, take this one week at a time. Reflect on your progress each week, adjusting your action plan as needed or adding new plans (over time, your current action plans will become habits, and you won't have to think about them as much). Use the following template to guide you.

Notice that this plan is behavior-based, and sets you up for building a healthy habit: in this case, walking for 30 minutes, 5 days per week. It also asks you to think of the challenges you might face ahead of time, so you have a plan for what to do if an excuse to not follow through comes up (such as bad weather, in the example above).

ACTION PLAN

BETWEEN _____ (DATE) AND _____ (DATE),

MY GOAL IS TO _____.

I will do this by:	Done? ○
Where will I do it?	
When will I do it?	
For how long will I do it?	
What challenges might I face?	
How will I overcome these challenges?	

ACTION PLAN (EXAMPLE)

BETWEEN _____January 6_____ (DATE) AND _____January 12_____ (DATE),

MY GOAL IS TO __be more active_____.

I will do this by:	Walking more · Done? ☑
Where will I do it?	My neighborhood
When will I do it?	At lunchtime, Monday through Friday
For how long will I do it?	30 minutes at a time
What challenges might I face?	Bad weather—cold, rain
How will I overcome these challenges?	Utilize a YouTube walking video or my Walking Pad

TIPS FOR CREATING ACTIONABLE GOALS

Make it realistic. Plan small changes that are realistic for you. Small changes have big effects over time. For example, including a vegetable in two meals per day may not sound like much, but when it's part of your daily routine, it adds up to a healthy habit that makes a big difference.

Be specific. What actions do you intend to do? Where, when, and for how long will you do them? For instance, if you plan to do more walking, for how long will you walk, and on how many days per week? Where will you do it, and how will you react if a challenge comes up?

Be flexible. Review your action plan each week, assessing what went well and what didn't. Look for ways to cope with challenges. If your plan isn't working for you, revise it. For example, if you made an action plan to walk in the mornings before work for 30 minutes, and you did not meet your goal, reflect on why. Perhaps you're not a morning person? Do you need to set an alarm to make sure you wake up 30 minutes earlier? Or do you need to adjust your plan and walk after work or at lunchtime instead, because walking in the morning simply isn't realistic for you?

Focus on behaviors. Change doesn't happen when you focus on the finish line. What actions can you take to reach that finish line? What behaviors need to change to allow you to reach your goal? You have control of your choices and actions. You can achieve the outcomes you want.

Make it enjoyable. Change doesn't need to be painful. Find foods and activities that you enjoy, and never focus on restricting yourself. Always think positively: What can I do instead of eating cookies at night? What can I add to my bedtime snack that would make it better? Can I replace my bedtime snack with another healthy habit?

ACTION STEPS FOR REDUCING INSULIN RESISTANCE

In chapter 1, we discussed four categories of lifestyle change that will help you reach the goal of reducing insulin resistance. Below, I'll explain how to put those changes into action in your own life. These simple, actionable steps are comprised of behaviors and habits that you can focus on to achieve remission of insulin resistance and improve your metabolic health in general. Remember: You don't have to do them all. These are simply examples, not a list you have to check off each week.

Incorporate regular physical activity into your day

- 30 minutes of walking daily
- Strength exercise: 2 to 3 times per week
- HIIT exercise: 1 to 3 times per week
- Recover with gentle yoga or stretching: 1 to 2 times per week

Prioritize sleep

- Get 7 to 9 hours of sleep hours every night
- Improve your sleep quality by creating a healthy bedtime routine
- Contact your doctor if you have chronic difficulty sleeping

Focus on stress management

- Reduce stress where possible

- Build healthy coping skills to manage stress, such as practicing meditation, mindfulness, and gratitude, or engaging in hobbies that bring you joy

- Limit your caffeine intake

- Limit your exposure to social media and news

Eat a balanced, nutrient-dense diet

- Eat a balanced diet comprised of healthy carbohydrates, lean proteins (both animal- and plant-based), nonstarchy vegetables, and foods that are rich in omega-3 fatty acids

- Emphasize high-fiber foods

- Reasonably limit foods that are high in saturated fat, sodium, refined carbohydrates, and added sugar.

By now, you know what insulin resistance is and the strategies that are important for reaching remission. You also know how to put that knowledge into action to transform your health. Your kitchen is stocked, your meal planning skills are strong, and you're ready to make changes. The most important part of this cookbook is, of course, the recipes. From breakfast to dinner and everything in between, each recipe in the following pages shows you how to apply what you've learned to make delicious, satisfying, insulin-friendly meals. Let's eat!

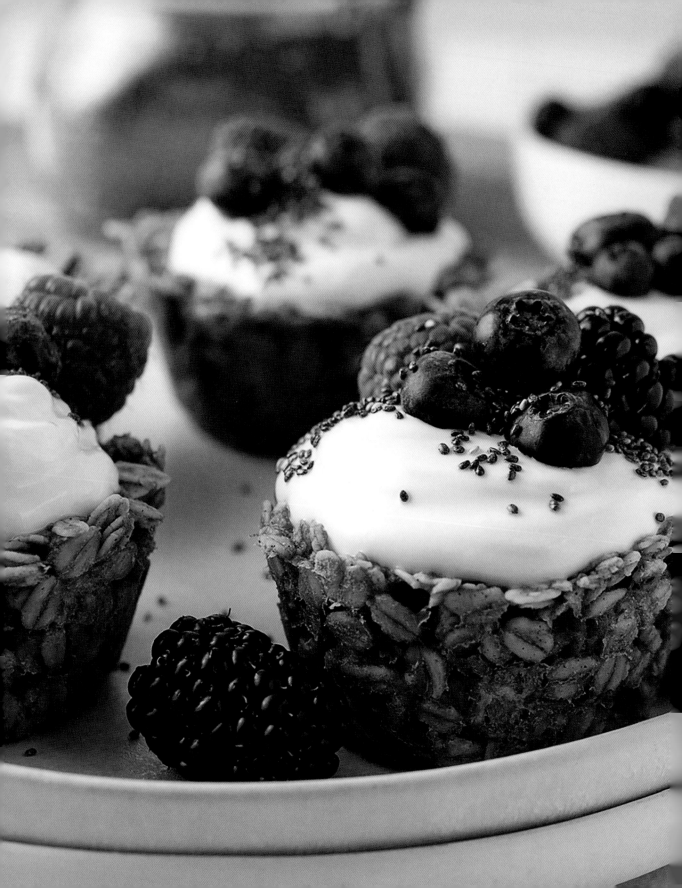

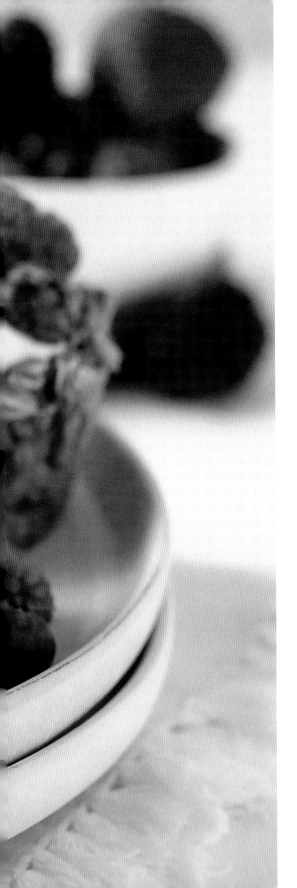

CHAPTER 3

15 Breakfasts in 15 Minutes

I know it's a bit of a cliché, but breakfast probably is the most important meal of the day for most people, especially if you have insulin resistance or another metabolic condition. Breaking your fast in the morning with a high-protein, high-fiber meal is a must when it comes to maintaining stable blood glucose and insulin levels throughout the day. The recipes in this chapter are here to help you do just that, even when life gets busy and rushed.

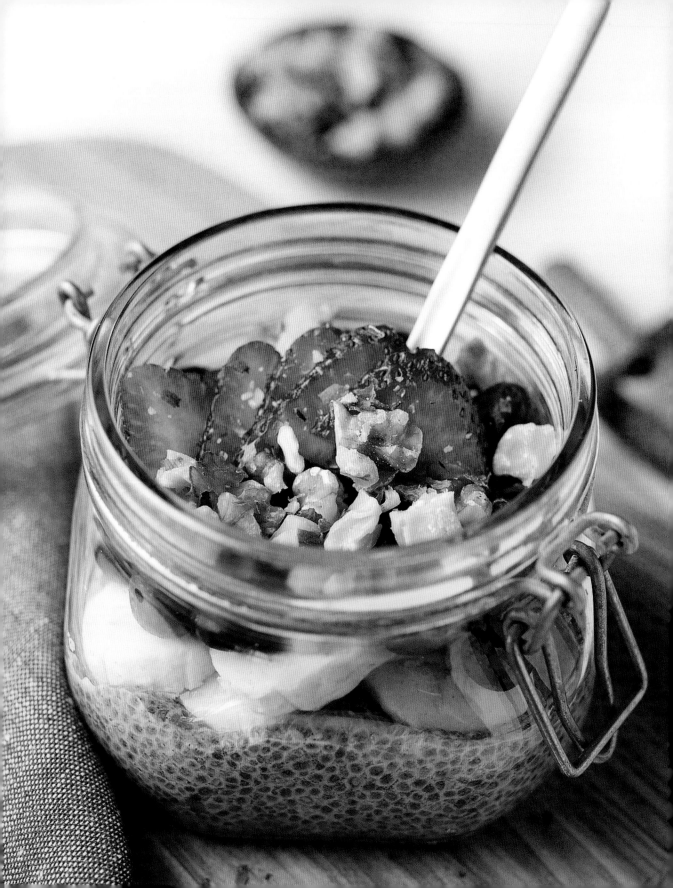

CHIA BLISS BOWL

This easy, make-ahead breakfast is full of key nutrients that improve insulin sensitivity, including fiber, protein, unsaturated fats, and magnesium. That's because chia seeds are little powerhouses of fiber and healthy fats, making them an ideal addition to smoothies, cereal, baked goods, and more.

YIELD:
1 SERVING

PREP TIME:
5 MINUTES

CHILL TIME:
4 HOURS OR
OVERNIGHT

3 tablespoons (45 g) chia seeds

¼ teaspoon ground cinnamon

⅔ cup (160 ml) almond milk

1 teaspoon sugar-free maple-flavored syrup

2 tablespoons (15 to 20 g) chopped nuts of your choice, such as walnuts or pecans

¼ cup (40 g) berries of your choice, such as blueberries or raspberries

½ banana, sliced

Optional toppings: other fruits, coconut flakes, sugar-free chocolate chips, and so on

Combine the chia seeds and cinnamon in a glass jar and gently shake to mix. Add the almond milk and maple-flavored syrup and mix well. Cover and refrigerate for at least 4 hours, or overnight.

Before serving, add the nuts, berries, banana, and optional toppings as desired.

NOTES

- **Tips:** Let the chia mixture sit for 5 minutes after combining, then give it one more good stir before you put it in the refrigerator. This will keep the chia seeds from clumping together. Or, for a smoother, pudding-like texture, you can combine the chia seeds, cinnamon, almond milk, and sweetener in a single-serve blender and pulse. This version also makes a delicious dessert.

- **Easy Swaps:** Feel free to swap the sugar-free maple-flavored syrup with your preferred liquid sweetener.

NUTRITIONAL ANALYSIS

SERVINGS SIZE: 1 jar

PER SERVING: 447 calories; 28 g fat; 12 g protein; 43 g carbohydrates; 20 g fiber

PREP-AHEAD OAT BOWLS WITH YOGURT AND BERRIES

Boost your weekday breakfast with these protein-packed oat bowls. Prep ahead for a 5-minute meal. The banana's sugar is balanced by fiber and protein!

▦ **YIELD:**
6 SERVINGS

▦ **PREP TIME:**
20 MINUTES

▦ **COOK TIME:**
45 MINUTES

▦ **ASSEMBLY TIME:**
5 MINUTES

FOR THE OAT BOWLS

2 medium bananas

¼ cup (60 ml) sugar-free maple-flavored syrup

½ cup (125 g) natural sugar-free peanut butter or nut butter of your choice

3½ cups (280 g) old-fashioned oats

¼ teaspoon salt

1 teaspoon ground cinnamon

FOR SERVING

1½ cups (360 g) plain or vanilla low-fat Greek yogurt

1 tablespoon (15 g) chia seeds or flax seeds

¾ cup (120 g) fresh berries

3 tablespoons (55 g) sugar-free chocolate chips (optional)

1 tablespoon (20 g) honey (optional)

Coat a standard 12-cup muffin pan with cooking spray, or use a silicone muffin pan.

Mash the bananas with a fork in a large mixing bowl. Add the maple-flavored syrup and nut butter and mix well. Add the oats, salt, and cinnamon and stir until evenly combined.

Scoop a heaping ¼ cup (about 55 g) of the mixture and drop into each cup in the muffin pan. Using a spoon and your fingers, press the mixture into the base and up the sides of the cups to create a hollow bowl shape (the sides of the mixture should extend slightly above the lip of each muffin cup).

Chill in the freezer for 30 minutes. Meanwhile, preheat the oven to 350°F (175°C).

Bake until set firm, 14 to 16 minutes. Firmly press the back of a spoon along the bottom and sides of each cup to solidify and reinforce the bowl shape. Let cool for 20 minutes. Gently remove the cups from the muffin pan and store in an airtight container.

To serve, into each cup add ¼ cup (60 g) yogurt, ½ teaspoon chia seeds, and 2 tablespoons (20 g) berries. Add 1½ teaspoons chocolate chips and ½ teaspoon honey, if using.

> **NOTES**
>
> - **Tip:** Try popping the oat bowls into the microwave for 20 seconds to warm them up before serving—a great contrast to the cool yogurt.
>
> - **Easy Swap:** To add 4 g of protein per serving, add 1 scoop (25 g) vanilla protein powder and 2 tablespoons (30 ml) milk to the oat bowl batter.

NUTRITIONAL ANALYSIS

SERVING SIZE: 2 oat cups with toppings

PER SERVING: 376 calories; 15 g fat; 13 g protein; 51 g carbohydrates; 9 g fiber

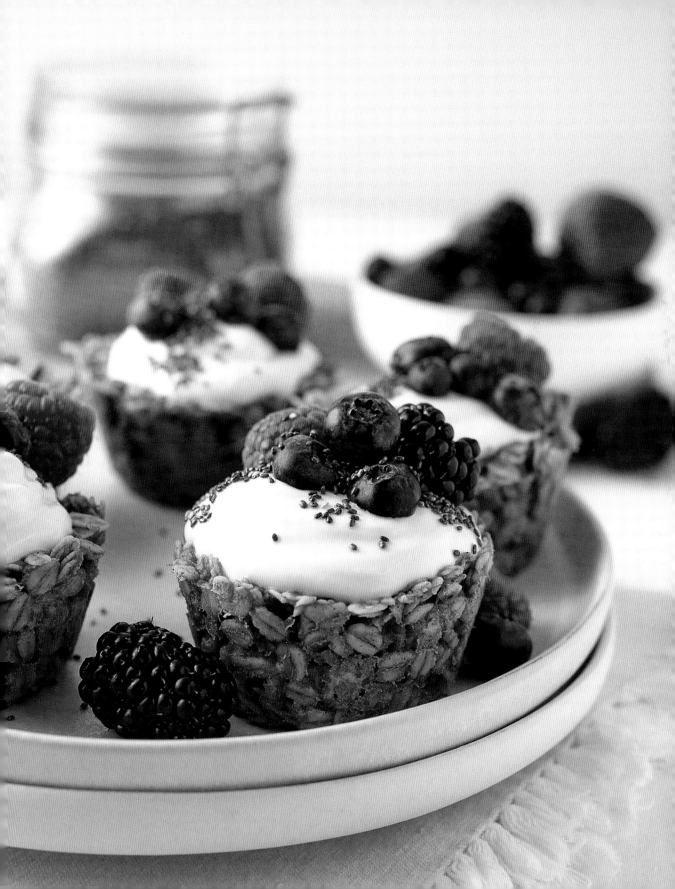

AVOCADO TOAST, THREE WAYS

YIELD:
1 SERVING

PREP TIME:
3 MINUTES

ASSEMBLY TIME:
2 MINUTES

Hearty, versatile avocado toast is so much more than a hipster trend. Avocados are a great addition to an insulin-friendly eating pattern. They're a surprisingly good source of fiber, with a whopping 6 grams per half of a medium-size avocado. The same amount of avocado also delivers 7 grams of healthy fats. Here are my three favorite ways to enjoy it.

FOR THE EGG & EVERYTHING SEASONING VERSION

1 slice whole-grain bread

½ medium-size avocado, pitted

2 large eggs, hard-boiled, peeled, and chopped

½ teaspoon everything but the bagel seasoning

FOR THE NUTTY VERSION

1 slice whole-grain bread

½ medium-size avocado, pitted

2 tablespoons (15 g) chopped walnuts

1 teaspoon whole flax seeds

FOR THE CAPRESE VERSION

1 slice whole-grain bread

½ medium-size avocado, pitted

Tomato slices

Splash of balsamic vinegar (a little goes a long way)

1 fresh basil leaf, coarsely chopped, or a sprinkle of dried basil

Light sprinkle of salt

NUTRITIONAL ANALYSIS (Egg & Everything Seasoning version)

SERVING SIZE: 1 toast

PER SERVING: 290 calories; 19 g fat; 16 g protein; 16 g carbohydrates; 7 g fiber

Toast the bread. Thinly slice the avocado while the flesh is still inside the skin. Using a spoon, scoop the flesh out of the peel and use a fork to mash it onto the toast.

Add your chosen toppings and dig in.

NOTES

- **Tips:** To pick the best possible avocado, give the avocado a gentle squeeze. It should have a little give, but shouldn't cave in. It should also be a dark green or brownish-green color. If you can only find avocados that are too hard to use right away, leave them to ripen on the counter for a few days or up to a week.

- **Easy Swap:** Try replacing the whole-grain bread with sourdough. It helps to support gut health and may enhance insulin sensitivity.

CHICKEN SAUSAGE SCRAMBLE WITH FRUIT AND TOAST

YIELD:
1 SERVING

PREP TIME:
5 MINUTES

COOK TIME:
8 MINUTES

Chicken sausage is a leaner alternative to most breakfast meats. It packs a punch of protein but has significantly less fat than most traditional pork sausages. Pair it with scrambled eggs and spinach and you've got a balanced breakfast with a whopping 30 grams of protein. Go ahead and add other veggies, if you like—no need to stop at spinach.

1 chicken apple sausage link

2 large eggs

½ cup (15 g) fresh spinach

1 slice whole-grain bread, toasted

½ cup (60 g) raspberries or other fruit of your choice

Place a small skillet over medium-high heat. Slice the sausage down the middle lengthwise, then chop into ½-inch (1.3 cm) thick pieces. Add to the skillet and cook until browned, about 5 minutes, stirring occasionally.

Meanwhile, place a medium skillet over medium heat. Coat with cooking spray, add the spinach, and cook, stirring occasionally so that the spinach begins to wilt. Crack the eggs into a small bowl and whisk, then add them to the skillet, stirring constantly with a silicone spatula for about 3 minutes, until cooked through and fluffy.

Add the cooked chicken sausage to the egg and spinach mixture. Transfer to a plate and serve immediately with a slice of whole-grain toast and berries.

NUTRITIONAL ANALYSIS

SERVING SIZE: 1 scramble, berries, toast

PER SERVING: 340 calories; 16 g fat; 30 g protein; 23 g carbohydrates; 7 g fiber

NOTES

- **Tip:** A quick note on sodium: Chicken sausage has a relatively high sodium content, but that doesn't mean you should blacklist it. Instead, assess your eating pattern over the whole day to make sure that your other meals aren't too high in sodium. It's all about balance, so it's okay to include some high-sodium foods.

- **Easy Swaps:** Try different flavors of your favorite chicken sausage, or replace with your preferred low-fat variety, such as turkey or veggie.

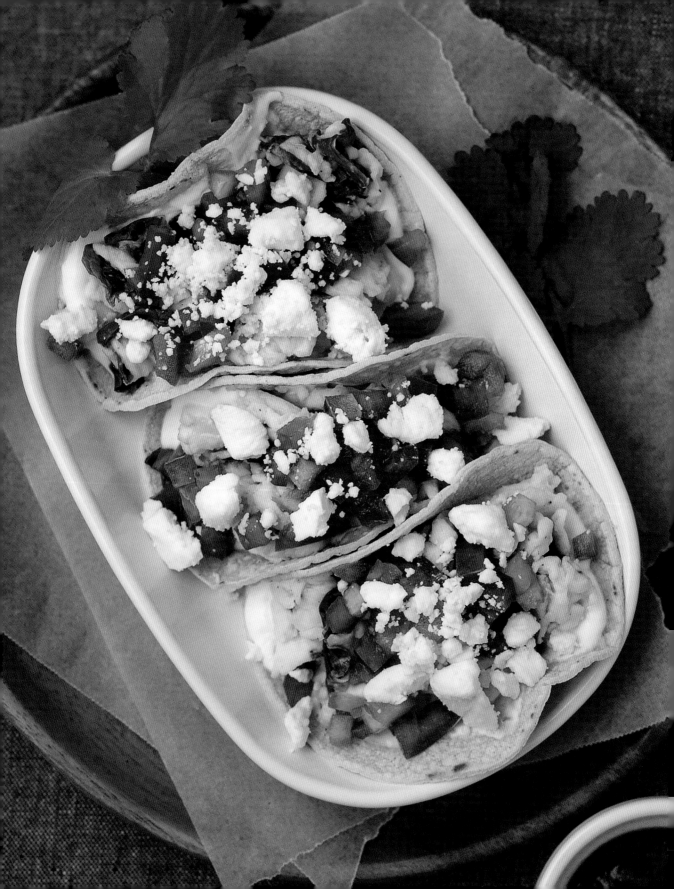

INSULIN-FRIENDLY BREAKFAST TACOS

Breakfast burritos can take a hike. These vegetarian tacos are even faster and easier to make. I like to make mine with corn tortillas, which are minimally processed and have tons of fiber, making them more wholesome than white-flour tortillas. Feel free to swap the corn tortillas for whole-wheat tortillas if you like, though.

▨ **YIELD:**
1 SERVING

▨ **PREP TIME:**
5 MINUTES

▨ **COOK TIME:**
5 MINUTES

▨ **ASSEMBLY TIME:**
2 MINUTES

3 large eggs

Salt and black pepper

¼ cup (10 g) chopped or torn greens, such as spinach or lettuce

3 4-inch (10 cm) corn tortillas

3 tablespoons (45 g) plain nonfat Greek yogurt

1 Roma tomato, diced

2 tablespoons (30 g) soft goat cheese

Hot sauce (optional)

Beat the eggs in a bowl with salt and pepper. Coat a small skillet with cooking spray and place over a medium heat. When hot, pour the eggs into the skillet and cook, stirring constantly with a rubber spatula. When the eggs are almost ready, add the spinach and cook for an additional 1 minute, until the spinach is wilted and the eggs are cooked through.

Heat a separate small skillet over medium-high. Warm each tortilla in the skillet for about 30 seconds on each side.

Place 1 tablespoon (15 g) of the yogurt on each tortilla. Top each tortilla with one-third of the eggs, one-third of the tomato, and one-third of the goat cheese. Add hot sauce, if desired. Serve immediately.

NOTES

- **Tip:** You'll notice that in a few recipes in this book I use Greek yogurt in place of sour cream. That's because it adds the same great tang, plus a protein boost.

- **Easy Swap:** You can use kale instead of spinach or lettuce here: Just sauté it in a separate skillet with 1 teaspoon of oil or 1 teaspoon balsamic vinegar (one or the other, not both) as you're preparing your eggs and tomato. Kale is a hearty green, so you'll need to soften it by cooking it a bit longer.

NUTRITIONAL ANALYSIS

SERVING SIZE: 3 tacos

PER SERVING: 419 calories; 19 g fat; 31 g protein; 32 g carbohydrates; 5 g fiber

BAKED EGGS WITH KALE AND TOMATO SAUCE

YIELD:
4 SERVINGS

PREP TIME:
10 MINUTES

COOK TIME:
15 MINUTES

This is my pared-down version of shakshuka, a North African dish that's also popular in the Middle East. It's easy to make, with just a handful of ingredients, but it's big on flavor (not to mention protein and fiber). I use sourdough bread here because sourdough undergoes a fermentation process that gives it a lower glycemic index than other breads. It's better for regulating blood glucose and contains gut-healthy probiotics, too.

1 tablespoon (15 ml) olive oil

2 cups (250 g) chopped kale

¼ teaspoon black pepper

24-ounce jar (680 ml)
    no-sugar-added lower
    sodium red pasta sauce

8 large eggs

4 slices sourdough bread,
    toasted

Preheat the oven to 400°F (200°C).

Heat the oil in a 12-inch (30 cm) cast-iron skillet over medium heat. Add the kale and season with half the black pepper. Sauté for 2 minutes or until kale starts to soften, then stir in the pasta sauce and bring to a simmer.

Using a spoon, make 8 wells in the sauce and crack an egg into each well. Sprinkle the remaining black pepper over the eggs. Transfer the pan to the oven and bake until the egg whites are set, about 10 minutes.

Divide among four plates and serve with the sourdough for dipping. Alternatively, store in the fridge for up to 3 days and reheat as needed.

NOTES

- **Tips:** Is your cast-iron pan smaller or larger than 12 inches (30 cm)? Never fear: Just watch the eggs as they bake, as they may cook more slowly or quickly depending the depth of your pan. If you don't have a cast-iron pan, start the recipe in a skillet, then transfer the sauce to a preheated baking dish and crack the eggs into it. Place the pan back into the oven and continue as above.

- **Easy Swap:** Swap the kale for spinach and breakfast will be on the table even faster; spinach cooks a bit more quickly than kale.

NUTRITIONAL ANALYSIS

SERVING SIZE: 2 eggs with
1 cup (about 250 g) sauce
and 1 slice of toast

PER SERVING: 418 calories;
15 g fat; 22 g protein;
42 g carbohydrates; 4 g fiber

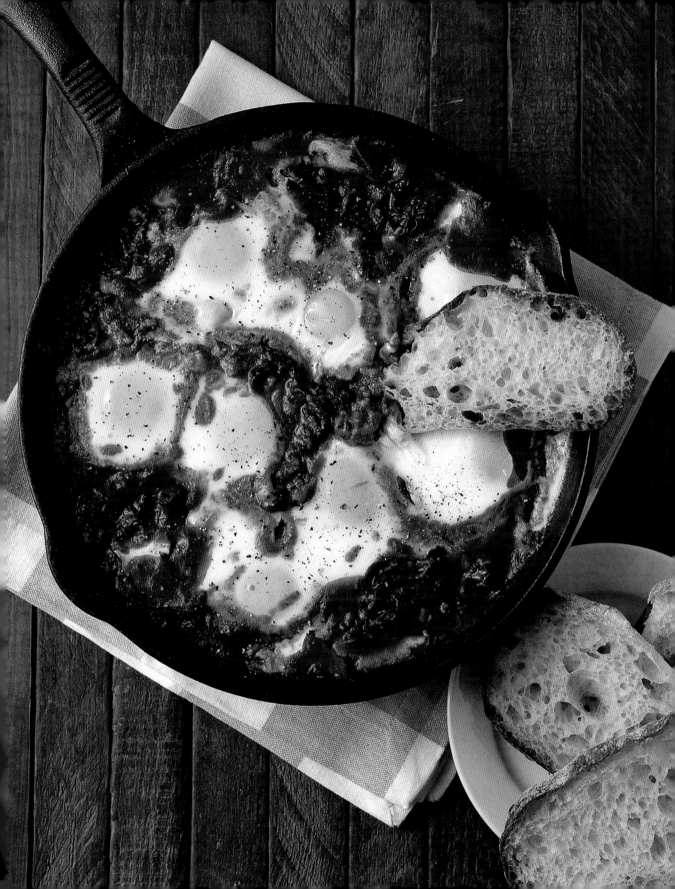

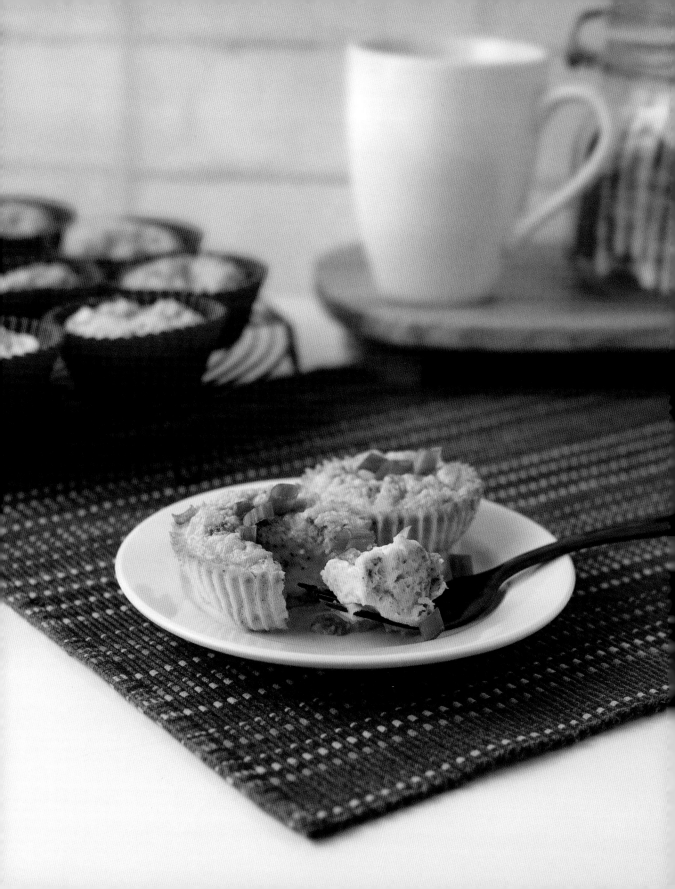

PREP-AHEAD CRUSTLESS MINI QUICHES

YIELD:
6 SERVINGS

PREP TIME:
10 MINUTES

COOK TIME:
14–18 MINUTES

These copycat egg bites take their inspiration from the wildly popular ones made by a certain coffeehouse chain. Pop them into the microwave for a 30-second breakfast solution on busy weekday mornings, and pair them with fruit or a slice of whole-grain toast.

10 large eggs

1 cup (225 g) low-fat cottage cheese

1 teaspoon hot sauce

1 cup (60 g) fresh spinach

1 Roma tomato, diced

½ cup (60 g) chopped sliced deli turkey

Optional ingredients: sliced mushrooms, chopped onion, or other veggies of your choice

Preheat the oven to 375°F (190°C). Coat a standard 12-cup muffin pan with cooking spray, or use a silicone muffin pan.

Blend the eggs, cottage cheese, and hot sauce in a food processor until smooth and airy, about 1 minute. Add the spinach and pulse four times, just until the spinach is finely chopped.

Divide the tomato and turkey among each of the muffin cups, followed by any of the optional toppings. Top each with an equal amount of the egg mixture, filling each cup about two-thirds full.

Bake for 14 to 18 minutes, until the mini quiches are set and don't wobble when you move the pan. Let cool for 5 minutes and enjoy immediately or cool and store in the fridge for up to 5 days. (Try making these on Sunday so breakfast is taken care of for the whole week.)

NOTES

- **Tips:** I love silicone muffin pans because you don't need to coat them with cooking spray. Make sure to set the silicone pan on top of a baking sheet before pouring in the liquid ingredients to keep the pan stable (I learned this the hard way...).

- **Easy Swaps:** Add more veggies or proteins (such as bell peppers, turkey bacon, diced ham, or black beans) to your mini quiches. More veggies mean more fiber. You can also swap my recommended toppings for your favorites. (Note that the nutrition analysis has been calculated with spinach, tomato and turkey, though.)

NUTRITIONAL ANALYSIS

SERVING SIZE: 2 mini quiches

PER SERVING: 150 calories; 8 g fat; 16 g protein; 4 g carbohydrates; 1 g fiber

EGG AND ARUGULA BREAKFAST SALAD

YIELD:
1 SALAD

PREP TIME:
3 MINUTES

COOK TIME:
4 MINUTES

ASSEMBLY TIME:
1 MINUTE

Growing up in the Midwest, I usually had the same breakfast most days: eggs, toast or oatmeal, fruit, maybe some bacon. Pancakes were served on weekends or holidays. But breakfast doesn't have to fit that mold. You're allowed to think outside the box and break your morning fast with a wholesome meal that isn't traditionally "breakfasty." When clients tell me that they're not breakfast people, I point them toward this savory salad.

2 large eggs

1 teaspoon avocado oil

⅛ teaspoon apple cider vinegar

⅛ teaspoon Dijon mustard

⅛ teaspoon sugar-free maple-flavored syrup

Pinch of salt

2 cups (60 g) packed arugula or fresh spinach

¼ cup (40 g) canned chickpeas, drained and rinsed

½ medium-size avocado, peeled, pitted, and sliced

1 teaspoon hemp seeds or flax seeds

Coat a small skillet with cooking spray and place over medium heat. Crack in the eggs and cook for about 3 minutes until the whites are set but the yolks remain runny, or to your preferred doneness.

Meanwhile, in a small bowl, whisk together the oil, vinegar, mustard, maple-flavored syrup, and salt to make a dressing.

Assemble the salad by arranging the eggs, greens, chickpeas, and avocado on a plate or in a shallow bowl. Top the with hemp seeds and the prepared dressing. Serve immediately.

NOTES

- **Tip:** This recipe doubles and even quadruples beautifully. You can make the dressing ahead of time if this salad is on the menu for several days running. It will last in the refrigerator for up to 4 days. Then simply prepare the rest of salad ingredients in a few minutes, and top with pre-made dressing.

- **Easy Swaps:** Chickpeas not your preferred pulse? Swap them with kidney beans, butter beans, or great northern beans. Hard-boiled eggs can replace fried eggs here, too.

NUTRITIONAL ANALYSIS

SERVING SIZE: 1 salad

PER SERVING: 530 calories; 32 g fat; 24 g protein; 3 g carbohydrates; 7 g fiber

HEARTY HARVEST BREAKFAST QUESADILLA

YIELD:
1 QUESADILLA

PREP TIME:
3 MINUTES

COOK TIME:
10 MINUTES

ASSEMBLY TIME:
1 MINUTE

I'm always really hungry in the morning. If you're like me, you might crave the kind of stick-to-your-ribs breakfast that'll keep you satisfied (and your blood sugar stable) until lunch time. Sound familiar? Look no further than this quick vegetarian quesadilla.

½ cup (15 g) fresh spinach

2 large eggs

Pinch of black pepper

¼ cup (40 g) canned black beans, rinsed and drained

2 tablespoons (30 g) chopped tomato

2 tablespoons (14 g) shredded cheddar cheese (optional)

1 8-inch (20 cm) Ole Xtreme high-fiber tortilla

1 tablespoon (15 g) plain nonfat Greek yogurt

1 tablespoon (15 g) salsa of choice

½ medium avocado, peeled, pitted, mashed with a fork

Coat a large skillet generously with cooking spray and place over medium heat. Add the spinach leaves and allow to wilt for about 2 minutes, then gently spread them out evenly in the skillet.

Meanwhile, beat the eggs and pepper in a medium bowl. Stir in the black beans and tomatoes. Add this mixture to the skillet, adding cheese, if using, and cook for 3 minutes. Gently lift the edge of the egg mixture with a rubber spatula and tilt the skillet to allow the uncooked egg from the top to run under the part that has already set.

Place the tortilla on top of the eggs in the pan and cook for 2 minutes more. When the eggs are fully cooked, carefully flip the entire quesadilla over and cook the other side of the tortilla for 1 minute.

Fold in half and cut outwards from the center of the flat edge into four wedges. Transfer to a plate, and serve with the Greek yogurt, salsa, and mashed avocado.

NOTES

- **Tips:** I love my toppings, so I add a mix of salsa, "sour cream" (that is, nonfat Greek yogurt), and mashed avocado to my quesadilla, but you can omit any or all of these. The nutrition facts here are calculated with Ole brand Xtreme high-fiber tortillas, and all three toppings.

- **Easy Swaps:** Substitute kale for spinach and any diced bell pepper for the tomatoes. You can also easily add your favorite veggies in addition to, or in place of, any of those used in this recipe. Use avocado slices instead of mashed avocado, if you like. If you can't find high-fiber tortillas, try whole-wheat tortillas.

NUTRITIONAL ANALYSIS

SERVING SIZE: 1 quesadilla

PER SERVING: 530 calories; 30 g fat; 34 g protein; 42 g carbohydrates; 22 g fiber

PROTEIN FRENCH TOAST WITH SPICED YOGURT TOPPING

■ **YIELD:**
4 SERVINGS

■ **PREP TIME:**
5 MINUTES

■ **COOK TIME:**
10 MINUTES

I don't often use protein powder in cooking because the best nutrition comes from whole foods, but this French toast is an exception. It is fluffy and high in protein and fiber, and makes great leftovers for fast weekday breakfasts. I like to crown it with a yogurt-based topping, but if that's not your speed, you can replace it with butter and sugar-free maple-flavored syrup.

FOR THE FRENCH TOAST

4 large eggs

½ cup (60 g) vanilla protein powder

½ cup (120 ml) 2% low-fat milk

½ teaspoon ground cinnamon

½ teaspoon pure vanilla extract

8 slices high-fiber bread

FOR THE SPICED YOGURT TOPPING

⅓ cup (80 g) nonfat plain Greek yogurt

1 tablespoon (15 ml) sugar-free maple-flavored syrup

⅛ teaspoon ground cinnamon

Pinch of ground nutmeg

Pinch of salt

To make the French toast, heat a griddle or skillet over medium heat.

In a large mixing bowl, whisk together the eggs, protein powder, milk, cinnamon, and vanilla. Dip each slice of bread into the egg mixture to coat generously.

Coat the hot griddle or skillet lightly with cooking spray, then arrange as many of the bread slices as will fit in a single layer without overlapping. Cook for about 3 minutes on each side, or until golden brown. Transfer to a plate to keep warm and repeat with the remaining bread slices.

To make the spiced yogurt topping, combine the yogurt, maple-flavored syrup, cinnamon, nutmeg, and salt in a small bowl and stir until well blended.

Serve the French toast immediately, topped with the spiced yogurt. Leftover French toast can be stored in the refrigerator for up to 4 days, or in an airtight container in the freezer for up to 6 months. Simply pop them in the toaster when you are ready to serve. Leftover yogurt can be stored in the refrigerator for up to 2 weeks.

NUTRITIONAL ANALYSIS

SERVING SIZE: 2 slices

PER SERVING: 248 calories; 6 g fat; 23 g protein; 28 g carbohydrates; 9 g fiber

NOTES

- **Tip:** Replace the spiced yogurt with toppings such as sugar-free chocolate chips, berries, butter, sugar-free maple-flavored syrup, or lightly sweetened whipped cream.
- **Easy Swap:** Make this recipe dairy-free by substituting your favorite plant-based milk and a coconut milk–based yogurt.

OVERNIGHT OATS, FOUR WAYS

■ YIELD:
1 SERVING

■ PREP TIME:
5 MINUTES

■ CHILL TIME:
6 HOURS TO
OVERNIGHT

Overnight oats are the ultimate weekday breakfast, but they also make a great snack. Don't be afraid of the high carb count: The fiber, good fats, and micronutrients in oats promote insulin sensitivity, so consuming these "good" carbs ultimately leads to reduced insulin resistance.

FOR THE CHOCOLATE OATS

½ cup (45 g) old-fashioned oats

½ cup (120 ml) 2% low-fat milk

⅓ cup (80 g) plain nonfat Greek yogurt

1½ teaspoons unsweetened cocoa powder

1 tablespoon (15 ml) sugar-free maple-flavored syrup or monk fruit sweetener

1 teaspoon chia seeds

Pinch of salt

Toppings: 1 tablespoon (15 g) sugar-free chocolate chips

FOR THE CARROT CAKE OATS

½ cup (45 g) old-fashioned oats

½ cup (120 ml) 2% low-fat milk

⅓ cup (80 g) plain nonfat Greek yogurt

2 tablespoons (20 g) shredded carrot

1 tablespoon (10 g) raisins

2 teaspoons (10 ml) sugar-free maple-flavored syrup or monk fruit sweetener

2 teaspoons (6 g) chopped walnuts

1 teaspoon chia seeds

½ teaspoon ground cinnamon

Pinch of ground ginger

Pinch of salt

FOR THE BANANA BERRY OATS

½ cup (45 g) old-fashioned oats

½ cup (120 ml) 2% low-fat milk

⅓ cup (80 g) plain nonfat Greek yogurt

2 teaspoons (10 ml) sugar-free maple-flavored syrup or monk fruit sweetener

1 teaspoon chia seeds

Pinch of salt

Toppings: ½ cup (60 g) sliced banana, ¼ cup (40 g) raspberries

NOTES

- **Tips:** Adjust the milk for your desired consistency. For a cozy, warm bowl, microwave the oats for 45 seconds.

- **Easy Swaps:** Try fun flavors like PB&J, apple-cinnamon, or pumpkin spice. Swap low-fat milk for plant-based options, but note the protein may be lower.

FOR THE TIRAMISU OATS

½ cup (45 g) old-fashioned oats

½ cup (120 ml) 2% low-fat milk

¼ cup (60 g) plain nonfat Greek yogurt

1 teaspoon instant coffee or espresso powder

1 teaspoon sugar-free maple-flavored syrup or monk fruit sweetener

¼ teaspoon pure vanilla extract

1 tablespoon (10 g) vanilla protein powder

1 teaspoon chia seeds

Pinch of salt

Topping: Dusting of ground cinnamon and unsweetened cocoa powder

For each variation, combine all the listed ingredients in a jar and stir well. Sprinkle with the toppings, if desired. Cover and refrigerate overnight or for a minimum of 6 hours.

NUTRITIONAL ANALYSIS (Chocolate Oats variation)

SERVING SIZE: 1 jar

PER SERVING: 474 calories; 12 g fat; 26 g protein; 65 g carbohydrates; 13 g fiber

WHIPPED TOFU AND BLUEBERRY COMPOTE ON TOAST

Think you don't like tofu? Well, this breakfast will change your mind. Whipped tofu is fluffy, slightly sweet, and filling, and it's a wonderful source of vegan protein. The luscious berry compote adds antioxidants and fiber but has no added sugar, making this an ideal insulin-friendly breakfast.

■ **YIELD:**
3 SERVINGS

■ **PREP TIME:**
5 MINUTES

■ **COOK TIME:**
10 MINUTES

■ **ASSEMBLY TIME:**
5 MINUTES

FOR THE COMPOTE

1½ cups (225 g) blueberries

2 tablespoons (30 ml) sugar-free maple-flavored syrup

1 tablespoon (15 ml) water

2 teaspoons (10 ml) lemon juice

1 teaspoon pure vanilla extract

FOR THE WHIPPED TOFU

1 (7 ounce/200 g) block firm tofu

1 tablespoon (15 ml) sugar-free maple-flavored syrup

2 teaspoons (10 ml) lemon juice

1 teaspoon pure vanilla extract

1 tablespoon (15 ml) 2% low-fat milk

¼ teaspoon lemon zest

⅛ teaspoon ground cinnamon

Pinch of salt

FOR SERVING

3 slices whole-grain bread

1 teaspoon lemon zest

NUTRITIONAL ANALYSIS

SERVING SIZE: 1 slice toast, ¼ cup (60 g) whipped tofu, 2 tablespoons (40 g) compote

PER SERVING: 176 calories; 4 g fat; 10 g protein; 23 g carbohydrates; 4 g fiber

To make the compote, combine the blueberries, maple-flavored syrup, water, lemon juice, and vanilla in a small saucepan and place over medium heat. Let the mixture cook and reduce for about 10 minutes, stirring frequently, until sauce has thickened to a syrupy consistency. Remove from the heat and set aside.

To make the whipped tofu, press the tofu to remove excess water (see page 30). Combine the pressed tofu, maple-flavored syrup, lemon juice, vanilla, milk, lemon zest, cinnamon, and salt in a food processor and blend for about 20 seconds. Scrape down the sides of the food processor and blend for another 20 seconds. Blend the mixture for 1 minute more, to incorporate plenty of air so that it's nice and fluffy.

To serve, toast the bread, then spread generously with the whipped tofu. Top each slice with one third of the compote and lemon zest. Store the prepared whipped tofu in the fridge for up to 2 days, and compote for up to 5 days.

NOTES

- **Tip:** If you're feeling fancy, add the tofu mixture to a pastry bag or a plastic storage bag with a ½-inch (1.3 cm) hole cut from the corner. Then squeeze onto your toast for a cool cake-icing look.

- **Easy Swaps:** Maple-flavored monk fruit sweetener works beautifully in this recipe in place of standard sugar-free maple-flavored syrup. No lemon on hand? Replace the lemon zest with orange zest.

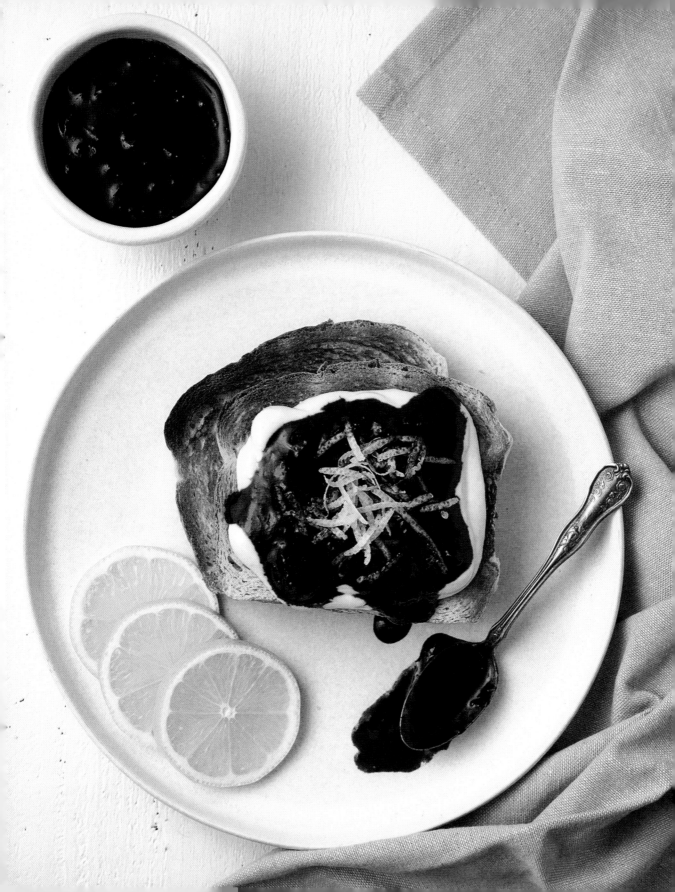

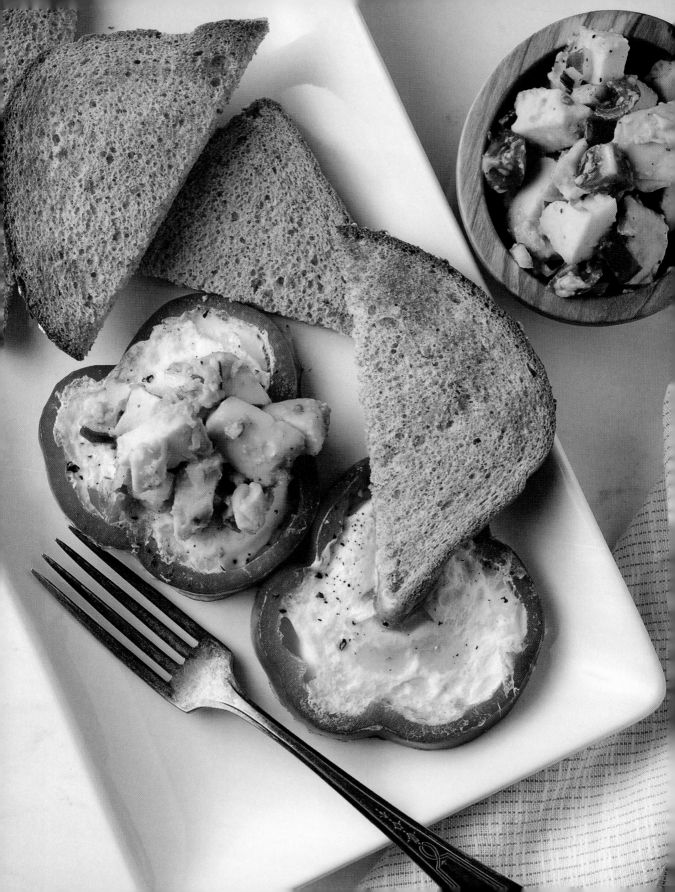

PEPPER-RING EGGS WITH FRESH AVOCADO SALSA

YIELD:
1 SERVING

PREP TIME:
5 MINUTES

COOK TIME:
5 MINUTES

As a kid, my family made a recipe that we called "egg with a hat." We'd cut a hole in a slice of bread and fry the egg in the hole, placing the cutout bread over the egg as its "hat." Now that I'm a dietitian, I wanted to create a version that would allow my insulin-resistant clients to control their carbs while delivering a dose of fiber-rich veggies. This fun, colorful breakfast is the result. Serve with a slice of whole-grain or sourdough toast or a serving of fruit.

1 red bell pepper

2 large eggs

Salt and black pepper

½ medium-size avocado, peeled, pitted, and diced

3 cherry tomatoes, diced

1 teaspoon diced red onion

¼ to ½ teaspoon lime juice

Slice off the top of the red pepper and remove the stem. Carefully slice around the core of the pepper and remove it. Cut the pepper into rings ½ inch (1.3 cm) thick. You will need two rings per serving.

Coat a medium (8-inch/20 cm) skillet with cooking spray and place over medium heat. Place the pepper rings in the skillet, then crack the eggs into them. Season with salt and pepper. Cook until the whites are almost set, about 2 minutes.

Meanwhile, prepare your avocado salsa. Combine the avocado, cherry tomatoes, onion, and lime juice in a small bowl. Season with salt and pepper and mix gently.

Flip the pepper-ringed eggs and continue to cook until yolk reaches desired doneness, about 1 minute. Transfer to a plate and top with the avocado salsa.

NOTES

- **Tips:** Remember that every person has unique nutrition needs. Consider adding carbohydrates to this meal in the form of toast or fruit, and in the amount that works best for you. For a larger serving size (and more protein), add an extra pepper-ring egg to your skillet.

- **Easy Swap:** Red not your favorite color? No problem: Swap the red bell pepper for yellow, orange, or green.

NUTRITIONAL ANALYSIS

SERVING SIZE: 2 eggs, ⅓ cup (80 ml) avocado salsa

PER SERVING: 265 calories; 19 g fat; 14 g protein; 10 g carbohydrates; 6 g fiber

PREP-AHEAD BAKED OATMEAL

YIELD:
8 SERVINGS

PREP TIME:
15 MINUTES

COOK TIME:
40 MINUTES

This gently spiced breakfast dish is the best way to start a weekend morning, but you can also make it ahead and enjoy it all week. I use a brown sugar baking blend here because it can be substituted 1 to 1 for sugar in any recipe with no effect on the recipe's structure, and no glycemic effect, either. Serve with a generous dollop of Greek yogurt.

3 cups (240 g) old-fashioned oats

½ cup (95 g) brown sugar baking blend

2 tablespoons (20 g) chia seeds

2 teaspoons (8 g) baking powder

½ teaspoon salt

½ teaspoon ground cinnamon (optional)

1¼ cups (300 ml) 2% low-fat milk

3 large eggs

1 cup (240 g) plain nonfat Greek yogurt

1 teaspoon pure vanilla extract

1 (15-ounce/425 g) can peaches in fruit juice, drained, left whole

½ cup (75 g) blueberries

⅓ cup (40 g) pecan or walnut pieces

Preheat the oven to 350°F (175°C). Coat a 7 by 11-inch (18 by 28 cm) baking dish with cooking spray.

Combine the oats, brown sugar baking blend, chia seeds, baking powder, salt, and cinnamon, if using, in a large mixing bowl.

Combine the milk, eggs, Greek yogurt, and vanilla in a separate bowl and whisk to blend.

Add the wet ingredients to the dry ingredients and stir just until combined. Let the mixture sit for 5 minutes to allow the oatmeal to start soaking up the liquid.

Gently mix in the peaches and blueberries until evenly distributed. Transfer to the prepared baking dish, spread evenly, and top with the nuts. Bake, uncovered, for 40 minutes, or until the oatmeal is set and does not move when you wiggle the pan.

Cut into eight slices and serve warm. Store leftovers in the refrigerator for up to 5 days. Reheat in the microwave when you are ready to serve.

NOTES

- **Tip:** For a slightly sweeter result, add 2 to 4 tablespoons (30 to 60 ml) of sugar-free maple-flavored syrup to the wet ingredients.

- **Easy Swaps:** Swap the canned peaches for fresh ones when they're in season. Or replace them with pomegranate seeds for a fun red, white, and blue Fourth of July theme. (Practically any fruit will work well here.) If you don't have a 7 by 11-inch (18 by 28 cm) baking dish, use a 9-inch (23 cm) square one.

NUTRITIONAL ANALYSIS

SERVING SIZE: 1 slice

PER SERVING: 362 calories; 9 g fat; 14 g protein; 55 g carbohydrates; 7 g fiber

MUESLI BOWL WITH YOGURT AND BERRIES

YIELD:
1 SERVING

PREP TIME:
5 MINUTES

Muesli, a cousin of granola, is a whole food combination of oats, berries, and nuts. When paired with a high-protein food like Greek yogurt, the result is a quick, filling breakfast that'll help stabilize your blood sugar. Think of it as a next-level bowl of cereal.

¼ cup (40 g) muesli

¼ cup (60 ml) 2% low-fat milk (optional)

⅓ cup (80 g) plain nonfat Greek yogurt

½ cup (about 75 g) berries of your choice

Pour the muesli into a cereal bowl. Add the milk to soften the grains, if you like (if so, let the muesli sit for 5 minutes). Top with the Greek yogurt and berries and serve immediately.

NOTES

- **Tip:** You can make your own muesli by mixing together 2 parts oats, 1 part "mix-ins," such as raisins, slivered almonds, and/or flax seeds, and a pinch each of cinnamon and salt.

- **Easy Swap:** Swap the berries for any in-season fruit.

NUTRITIONAL ANALYSIS

SERVING SIZE: 1 bowl

PER SERVING: 220 calories; 10 g fat; 12 g protein; 20 g carbohydrates; 8 g fiber

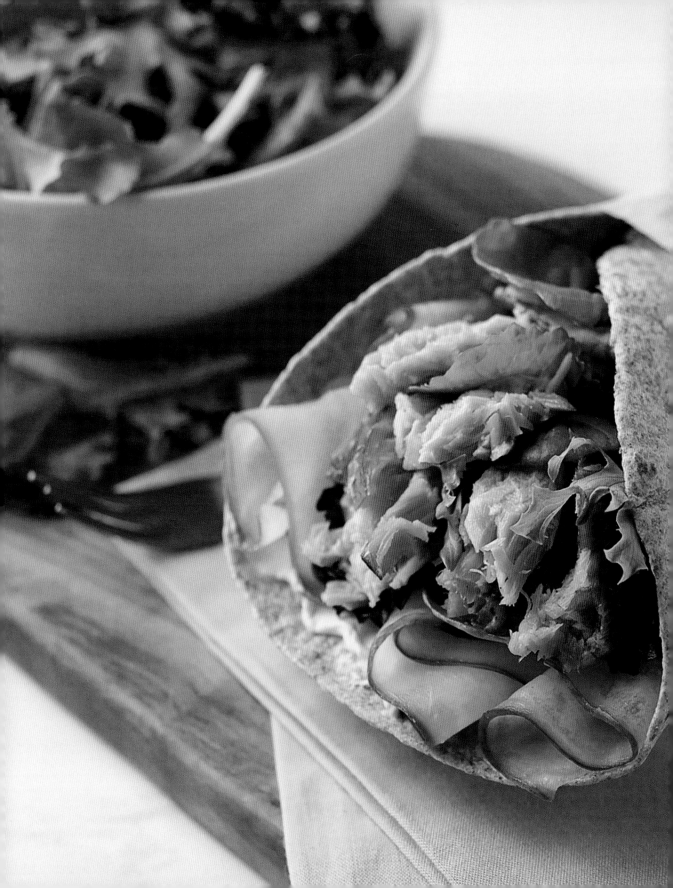

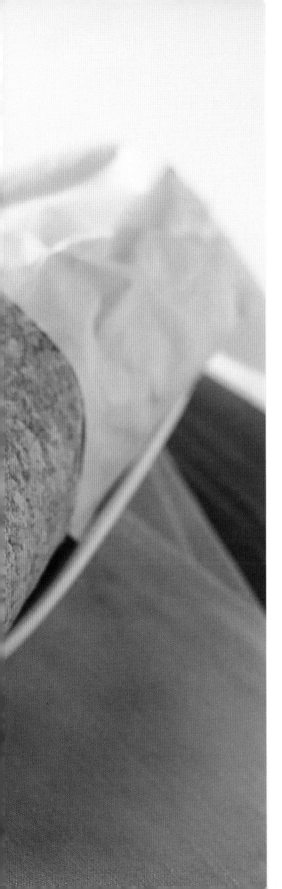

CHAPTER 4

15 Lunches in 15 Minutes

Most people are so busy at lunchtime that it slips past in the blink of an eye. But it's vital to take the time to eat a nutritious midday meal that will power you through the afternoon while keeping your blood sugar stable. The recipes in this chapter are quick, portable, easy to prep, and designed to make lunchtime a no-brainer—because you have more important things to think about.

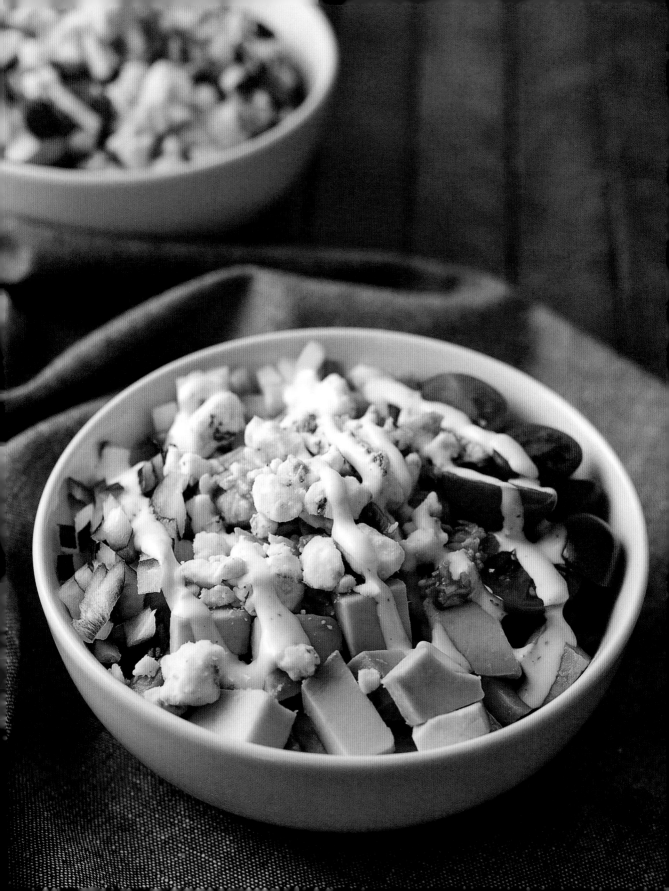

BUFFALO CHICKEN POWER BOWLS

Loaded with protein and fiber and bursting with bold flavors, this high-volume, ten-minutes-to-the-table meal will fuel you for the whole afternoon. You can use rotisserie chicken here, but preparing your own shredded chicken breasts ahead of time is preferable because rotisserie chicken tends to be higher in sodium. Either way, I have a hunch that this one will find its way onto your repeat list.

YIELD:
2 SERVINGS

PREP TIME:
5 MINUTES

COOK TIME:
5 MINUTES

ASSEMBLY TIME:
5 MINUTES

- 1 cup (100 g) frozen cauliflower rice
- 1 cup (185 g) uncooked microwaveable single-serve brown rice cup
- 2 cups (300 g) shredded cooked chicken
- ⅓ cup (80 ml) buffalo sauce
- ½ medium-size avocado, peeled, pitted, and diced
- ½ cup (80 g) cherry tomatoes, halved
- ¼ cup (40 g) diced red onion
- ¼ cup (40 g) diced celery
- ¼ cup (30 g) crumbled blue cheese
- 2 tablespoons (30 ml) ranch dressing

Add 1 tablespoon (15 ml) of water to the cauliflower rice, cover, and steam in the microwave for 3 minutes.

Microwave the rice according to package directions. Stir into the cauliflower rice and set the mixture aside.

Mix the chicken with buffalo sauce. Divide the rice mixture between two separate bowls. Top each with equal portions of the buffalo chicken, avocado, cherry tomatoes, red onion, celery, and blue cheese.

Drizzle each bowl with ranch dressing and serve.

NOTES

- **Tips:** Microwaveable single-serve rice cups are perfect for this quick lunch. If you can't find cauliflower rice, you can make your own in less than a minute by placing cauliflower florets in a food processor and pulsing approximately 10 times.

- **Easy Swaps:** For a plant-based protein, switch out the chicken for tofu or tempeh. Also, remember that everyone's carbohydrate needs are unique, so if you need more carbs, replace the cauliflower rice with basmati rice or double the brown rice.

NUTRITIONAL ANALYSIS

SERVING SIZE: 1 bowl

PER SERVING: 513 calories; 28 g fat; 60 g protein; 14 g carbohydrates; 4 g fiber

CHICKEN AND CUCUMBER GREEN GODDESS WRAP

■ **YIELD:**
1 SERVING

■ **PREP TIME:**
3 MINUTES

■ **ASSEMBLY TIME:**
2 MINUTES

My pared-back version of green goddess dressing really makes this quick, fiber-rich wrap stand out. Using cooked chicken means you can pull it together in just a couple minutes, so it's great for WFH days when you're squeezing in lunch between online meetings. If you aren't used to consuming a lot of fiber, increase your intake gradually and drink lots of water to avoid initial tummy discomfort.

¼ **medium-size avocado**

1 **tablespoon (15 g) whipped cream cheese**

1 **teaspoon lemon juice**

Salt and black pepper

1 **tablespoon (2 g) chopped fresh parsley or 1½ teaspoons dried**

1 **8-inch (20 cm) Ole Xtreme high-fiber tortilla**

¾ **cup (120 g) shredded cooked chicken breast**

¼ **cup (30 g) sliced cucumber**

Handful of greens (about 30 g), such as spinach, arugula, or lettuce

Mash the avocado in a small bowl. Stir in the cream cheese, lemon juice, and salt and pepper. Add the parsley and mix until well combined. Spread the mixture evenly on the tortilla. Add the chicken, cucumber, and greens. Roll up burrito-style and serve.

NOTES

- **Tip:** Save time by preparing the avocado mixture in advance and storing in an airtight container for up to 4 days.

- **Easy Swaps:** No fresh herbs on hand? Swap out the fresh parsley with 1 teaspoon dried. To keep sodium to a minimum, prep your own chicken breast ahead of time (see page 30): It'll stay fresh in the refrigerator for up to 5 days. But if you're running short on time, rotisserie chicken will do the trick. Just keep an eye on your overall sodium intake for the day.

NUTRITIONAL ANALYSIS

SERVING SIZE: 1 wrap

PER SERVING: 398 calories; 19 g fat; 48 g protein; 20 g carbohydrates; 13 g fiber

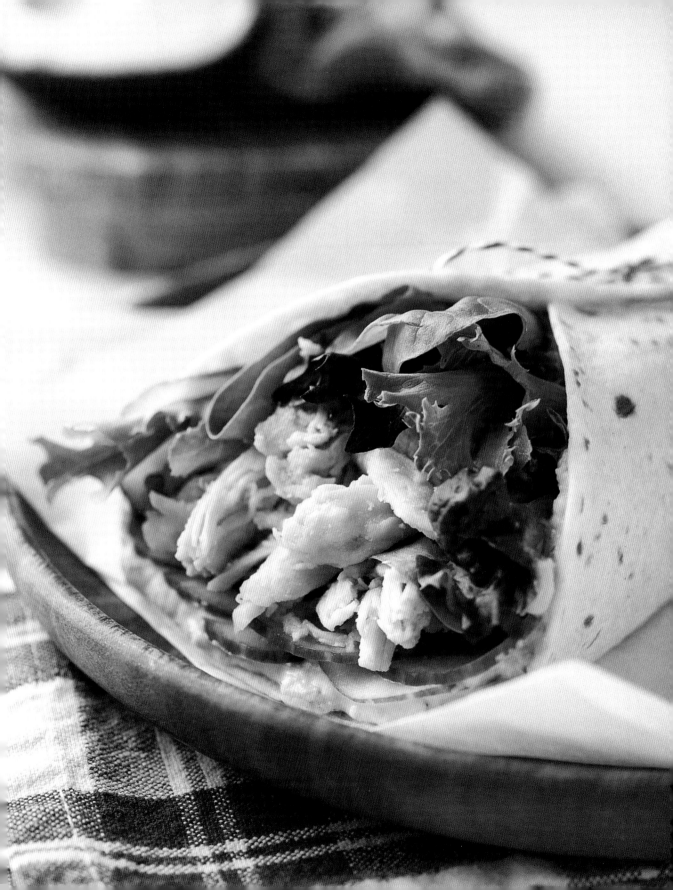

TURKEY MELT WITH TOMATO COMPOTE AND ARUGULA

■ **YIELD:**
1 SERVING

■ **PREP TIME:**
5 MINUTES

■ **COOK TIME:**
10 MINUTES

You don't have to strike sandwiches from the menu just because you're insulin resistant. This one features fiber sources and helps you hit your protein goal, so it's a very stabilizing meal. Use carved turkey (available in most grocery stores in the refrigerated deli meat section) instead of deli turkey: It's minimally processed in comparison.

FOR THE TOMATO COMPOTE
¼ teaspoon olive oil
½ cup (75 g) cherry tomatoes
¼ teaspoon balsamic vinegar

FOR THE SANDWICH
2 slices whole-grain bread
1 tablespoon (15 g) mayonnaise
3 ounces (85 g) carved turkey
1 slice Swiss cheese
½ cup (20 g) arugula

To make the tomato compote, combine the olive oil and whole cherry tomatoes in a small saucepan over medium heat. Cook until the tomatoes burst, about 5 minutes, then smash them gently with a spatula. Add the balsamic vinegar and stir. Remove from the heat and set aside until you are ready to serve.

To make the sandwich, heat a small skillet over medium heat. Spread half of the mayonnaise on one side of each slice of bread. Add one slice to the pan, mayo side down. Layer the turkey and cheese onto the bread and top with the second slice. Cook for about 3 minutes, flipping once, until both sides are golden brown.

Transfer the sandwich to a plate. Remove one slice of bread, spread with the tomato compote, top with arugula, then place the bread back on top and serve.

NOTES

- **Tips:** Skip the chips and serve this sandwich with ½ cup (75 g) crispy chickpeas (store-bought is fine) for a satisfying crunch. The tomato compote is delicious on avocado toast, as an addition to a salad, or even as another sandwich spread. You can double or triple the recipe and store in the refrigerator for up to 5 days if you'd like.

- **Easy Swap:** Baby spinach makes a nice substitute for arugula here.

NUTRITIONAL ANALYSIS

SERVING SIZE: 1 sandwich

PER SERVING: 393 calories;
22 g fat; 30 g protein;
19 g carbohydrates; 6 g fiber

GREENS AND BEANS TOMATO SOUP

This recipe was born when I wanted to create a wholesome meal out of a simple pleasure: store-bought tomato soup. It adds plant-based protein and fiber to the mix and is great for sick days or whenever you need a comforting, nutritious meal fast.

■ **YIELD:**
2 SERVINGS

■ **PREP TIME:**
2 MINUTES

■ **COOK TIME:**
10 MINUTES

1 (10-ounce/280 g) can condensed tomato soup

1 teaspoon olive oil

1½ cups (45 g) chopped kale

1 (15-ounce/400 g) can cannellini beans, rinsed and drained

2 tablespoons (15 g) grated Parmesan cheese

Sprinkle of dried red pepper flakes (optional)

Add water and heat the soup in a medium saucepan according to can directions. Simmer over low heat.

Meanwhile, heat the oil in a large skillet over medium heat. Add the kale and cook, stirring until wilted, 1 to 2 minutes. Add the kale and beans to the soup and simmer until the beans are heated through, 2 to 3 minutes.

Divide the soup between two bowls. Top each with 1 tablespoon (8 g) of the Parmesan cheese and a sprinkle of red pepper flakes, if using.

NOTES

- **Tip:** Canned tomato soup is high in sodium, so make sure to choose a low-sodium or unsalted version so you can control the amount you consume.

- **Easy Swaps:** Feel free to swap out the kale for spinach, or even chopped lettuce (if you've never tried this before, trust me: It works). If you are using lettuce, you do not need to wilt it in a separate skillet prior to adding to the soup.

NUTRITIONAL ANALYSIS

SERVING SIZE: 2 cups (475 ml)

PER SERVING: 269 calories; 6 g fat; 14 g protein; 43 g carbohydrates; 9 g fiber

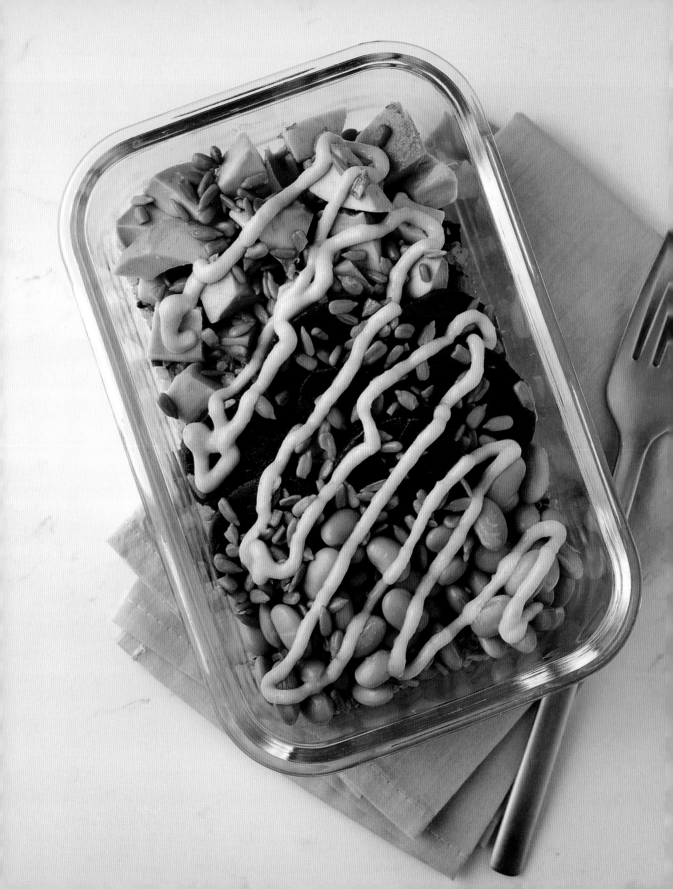

VEGAN GRAIN BOWLS

These grain bowls are proof that you can prep lunches for the entire week in just 10 minutes. They're perfect if you're eating on the go, or if your workplace has limited kitchen facilities, because there's no need to heat them up. Hummus and edamame are both great plant-based sources of protein, and research has shown that eating two servings of pulses (beans, peas, lentils, and chickpeas) per day can improve heart health, digestive health, weight management, and blood sugar control.

■ YIELD:
4 SERVINGS

■ COOK TIME:
5 MINUTES

■ ASSEMBLY TIME:
5 MINUTES

1 cup (185 g) uncooked microwaveable single-serve brown rice or quinoa cup

1 cup (240 g) hummus

2 tablespoons (30 ml) lemon juice

1 (5-ounce/140 g) package fresh baby kale or baby spinach

1 (8-ounce/225 g) package refrigerated cooked sliced beets

2 cups (300 g) frozen edamame, thawed

2 medium-size avocados, peeled, pitted, and diced

¼ cup (30 g) toasted or raw sunflower seeds or pine nuts

Prepare the quinoa or rice pouch according to the package directions and set aside.

Combine the hummus and lemon juice in a small bowl. Divide into four small condiment containers.

Divide the kale or spinach into four meal prep containers. Top each with ½ cup (90 g) prepared quinoa or rice, ½ cup (65 g) beets, ½ cup (80 g) edamame, ½ diced avocado, and 1 tablespoon (2 g) sunflower seeds or pine nuts.

When you are ready to serve, drizzle one portion of the hummus mixture on top of the grain bowl.

NOTES

- **Tip:** Sometimes shortcuts are worth it. It's fine to use microwavable grain pouches of rice or quinoa to speed up meal prep. I also keep a few on hand so that I have a nutritious, high-fiber base for meals on especially busy days.

- **Easy Swaps:** If you don't like beets, replace them with pickled carrots or your favorite roasted veggies.

NUTRITIONAL ANALYSIS

SERVING SIZE: 1 bowl

PER SERVING: 335 calories; 24 g fat; 20 g protein; 13 g carbohydrates; 6 g fiber

CUCUMBER, CRAB, AND AVOCADO SUSHI ROLLS

■ **YIELD:**
2 SERVINGS

■ **PREP TIME:**
5 MINUTES

■ **ASSEMBLY TIME:**
5 MINUTES

This lower-carb take on a sushi roll keeps the focus on protein and fiber, unlike traditional sushi, which runs heavy on the rice. It's still a balanced meal, though, thanks to the carbohydrate in imitation crab. If you need additional carbs to meet your personal needs, add a side of fruit.

8 ounces (225 g) flake-style imitation crab

¼ cup (60 g) low-fat plain Greek yogurt

1 teaspoon Dijon mustard

1 teaspoon lemon juice

2 tablespoons (10 g) chopped green onions, light and dark green parts only

1 teaspoon chopped fresh parsley, or ½ teaspoon dried

Salt and black pepper

1 cucumber

½ cup (120 g) whipped cream cheese

1 medium-size avocado, peeled, pitted, and sliced

In a mixing bowl, combine the crabmeat, yogurt, Dijon mustard, lemon juice, green onions, and parsley. Season to taste with salt and pepper. Stir until well combined and set aside.

Using a vegetable peeler, slice the cucumber lengthwise into long, thin ribbons. The first and last slices will be mostly peel: Discard these, as they're too thick to roll smoothly.

Lay eight cucumber ribbons on a clean paper towel vertically, slightly overlapping so that they form a continuous "sheet." Pat the cucumber ribbons dry with another paper towel to remove excess moisture.

Spread 2 tablespoons (30 g) of whipped cream cheese evenly across the cucumber ribbons. Next, arrange one-quarter of the avocado slices in a neat vertical line about an inch from the left edge of the cucumber sheet. Spoon one-quarter of the crab mixture onto the cucumber slices right beside the avocado.

Starting from the left side, carefully roll the cucumber ribbons over the fillings, keeping the roll tight and firm to create a "sushi" roll. Repeat the process with the remaining ingredients to make a total of four rolls. To serve, gently slice each roll into bite-sized sushi-style pieces.

NOTES

- **Tip:** If you're using chunk-style imitation crab, make sure to chop or tear it into smaller pieces before making the crab salad.

- **Easy Swaps:** You could swap the crab salad filling for sushi-grade salmon or other fish, or the chicken salad on page 73.

NUTRITIONAL ANALYSIS

SERVING SIZE: 2 rolls

PER SERVING: 381 calories; 21 g fat; 17 g protein; 23 g carbohydrates; 2 g fiber

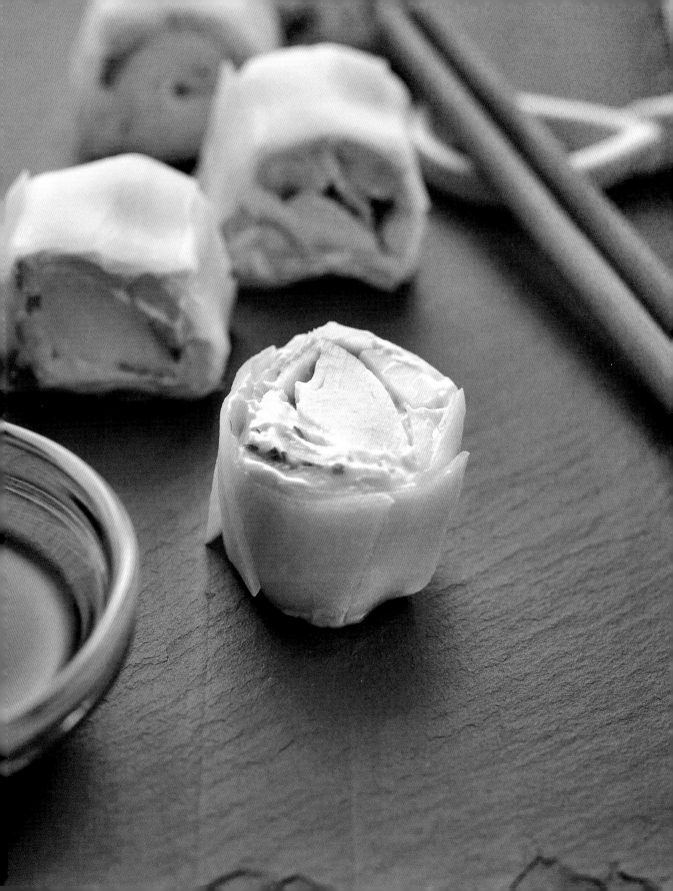

TUNA AND BEAN–STUFFED AVOCADOS

■ YIELD:
2 SERVINGS

■ PREP TIME:
5 MINUTES

You can't beat avocado and tuna if you're looking to up your intake of healthy fats. Add some black beans, and you've got a well-balanced, no-cook, insulin-friendly lunch. This meal also does double-duty as an afternoon snack if you've got a late dinner planned and you're already starving. Serve with a couple handfuls of crispy chickpeas, if you like.

2 avocados

⅓ cup (80 g) plain nonfat Greek yogurt

¼ cup (30 g) finely chopped celery

½ cup (30 g) finely chopped fresh spinach

1 cup (170 g) cooked black beans, drained and rinsed

2 packs (5.2 ounces/147 g) flavored tuna

1 teaspoon hemp seeds (optional)

Slice the avocados lengthways and remove the pit, leaving the flesh attached to the skin.

Combine the yogurt, celery, spinach, beans, and tuna in a bowl. Stuff and top the avocado halves with the tuna mixture and sprinkle each with hemp seeds.

NOTES

- **Tip:** Using the halved avocadoes makes a lovely presentation, but you can also serve the tuna mixture in a bowl and top with avocado slices or chunks.

- **Easy Swaps:** If you're using regular canned tuna instead, consider adding your own flavor combinations, like this Asian-inflected one: Add ground cumin, chili powder, white pepper, sriracha sauce, and a dash of salt to the tuna. Mix well, then proceed with the recipe.

NUTRITIONAL ANALYSIS

SERVING SIZE: 1 stuffed avocado

PER SERVING: 531 calories; 32 g fat; 36 g protein; 22 g carbohydrates; 7 g fiber

THE CHICKEN SALAD SALAD

Like the egg salad sandwiches on page 74, chicken salad sandwiches are deli classics. My version is a salad with added chickpeas for extra texture and fiber. Then I serve the whole thing on a bed of greens. Use whole-grain crackers for scooping.

■ **YIELD:**
3 SERVINGS

■ **PREP TIME:**
10 MINUTES

■ **ASSEMBLY TIME:**
1 MINUTE

2 cups (300 g) shredded cooked chicken

½ cup (80 g) canned chickpeas, drained and rinsed

½ cup (120 g) mayonnaise

¼ cup (30 g) chopped celery

¼ cup (40 g) chopped red onion

2 teaspoons (10 g) Dijon mustard

½ teaspoon garlic powder

⅛ teaspoon salt

⅛ teaspoon black pepper

6 cups (180 g) salad greens

2 Roma tomatoes, chopped

6 crispbreads or whole-grain crackers

Combine the chicken, chickpeas, mayonnaise, celery, red onion, mustard, garlic powder, salt, and pepper in a medium-size bowl and mix well.

Assemble the salads by placing 2 cups (60 g) of salad greens into each of three bowls, topping each with a chopped Roma tomato and 1 cup (150 g) of the chicken salad. Serve with crispbreads or whole-grain crackers.

NOTES

- **Tips:** Chickpeas add fiber, protein, and a nice texture. You can always use the chicken salad mixture on a sandwich if you need more carbohydrates at your meals and the crackers aren't enough. Alternatively, you could add a side of fruit to increase the carb content.

- **Easy Swap:** Swap out the tomatoes for other veggies, such as carrots, radishes, and so on.

NUTRITIONAL ANALYSIS

SERVING SIZE: 1 cup (150 g) chicken salad, 2 cups (60 g) salad veggies, 2 crispbreads

PER SERVING: 572 calories; 33 g fat; 33 g protein; 36 g carbohydrates; 8 g fiber

EGG SALAD SANDWICH

■ YIELD:
4 SERVINGS

■ PREP TIME:
10 MINUTES

Deli-style egg salad is a satisfying lunchtime staple, but when it's made with full-fat mayo, it can be a bit heavy. This version relies on Dijon mustard, green onions, and lemon zest for flavor and uses Greek yogurt for a light but creamy texture (and added protein and calcium).

FOR THE EGG SALAD

8 large eggs, hard-boiled, peeled, and chopped

⅓ cup (80 g) nonfat plain Greek yogurt

1½ teaspoons Dijon mustard

3 tablespoons (15 g) thinly sliced green onions, light and dark green parts only

⅓ cup (45 g) finely chopped celery

¼ teaspoon lemon zest

1 tablespoon (10 g) chopped fresh parsley or 1 teaspoon dried

½ teaspoon salt, or to taste

¼ teaspoon black pepper, or to taste

FOR SERVING

8 slices whole-grain bread, toasted

½ cup (90 g) tomato slices, or more or less to taste

1 cup (47 g) torn romaine lettuce, or more or less to taste

Chop the eggs and put in a large mixing bowl.

In a small bowl, whisk together the yogurt, mustard, green onions, celery, lemon zest, parsley, salt, and pepper. Add this mixture to the eggs and combine well. Adjust the seasoning if necessary.

Serve one-quarter of the mixture, topped with tomato slices and lettuce, between two slices of toasted whole-grain bread. Repeat to make four sandwiches.

NUTRITIONAL ANALYSIS

SERVING SIZE: 1 sandwich with ½ cup (110 g) egg salad

PER SERVING: 233 calories; 9 g fat; 20 g protein; 20 g carbohydrates; 5 g fiber

NOTES

- **Tips:** Egg salad is a great sandwich filler, but it can also be used as a dip for crackers or veggies. Or, spread it on toast and top it with avocado slices for a quick savory breakfast.

- **Easy Swap:** For a slightly tangier egg salad, swap the lemon zest for about ¼ teaspoon lemon juice.

ZESTY LEMON, SHRIMP, AND AVOCADO SALAD

■ YIELD:
4 SERVINGS

■ PREP TIME:
10 MINUTES

With its citrusy flavors and loads of fresh veggies, this shrimp salad makes a fabulous summer lunch, since you don't have to go anywhere near the stove to whip it up. Spoon it over a bed of quinoa or serve it alongside some fruit to add wholesome carbohydrates for a balanced meal.

1 pound (450 g) peeled cooked shrimp

1 large avocado, peeled, pitted, and diced

1½ cups (225 g) halved cherry tomatoes

1 stalk celery, diced

2 green onions, light and dark green parts only, sliced

¼ cup (15 g) coarsely chopped fresh cilantro

1 tablespoon (15 ml) avocado oil

1 teaspoon minced garlic

2 tablespoons (30 ml) fresh lemon juice

½ teaspoon lemon zest

Salt and black pepper

¼ cup (28 g) crumbled feta cheese, for serving

Remove the tails from the shrimp, if necessary, and chop each into approximately three bite-size pieces. Combine the chopped shrimp, avocado, cherry tomatoes, celery, green onions, and cilantro in a large bowl. Stir gently until well mixed. Add the oil, garlic, lemon juice, and zest. Season to taste with salt and pepper.

Serve immediately, or cover and refrigerate for an hour to let the flavors marry. When you are ready to serve, top each serving of shrimp salad with 1 tablespoon (7 g) of feta cheese. Store in an airtight container for up to 3 days.

NUTRITIONAL ANALYSIS

SERVING SIZE: 1 cup (190 g)

PER SERVING: 218 calories; 13 g fat; 19 g protein; 2 g carbohydrates; 2 g fiber

NOTES

- **Tip:** This recipe also makes a great appetizer for a party or potluck.

- **Easy Swap:** Lots of people dislike cilantro. If you're one of them, swap it with parsley.

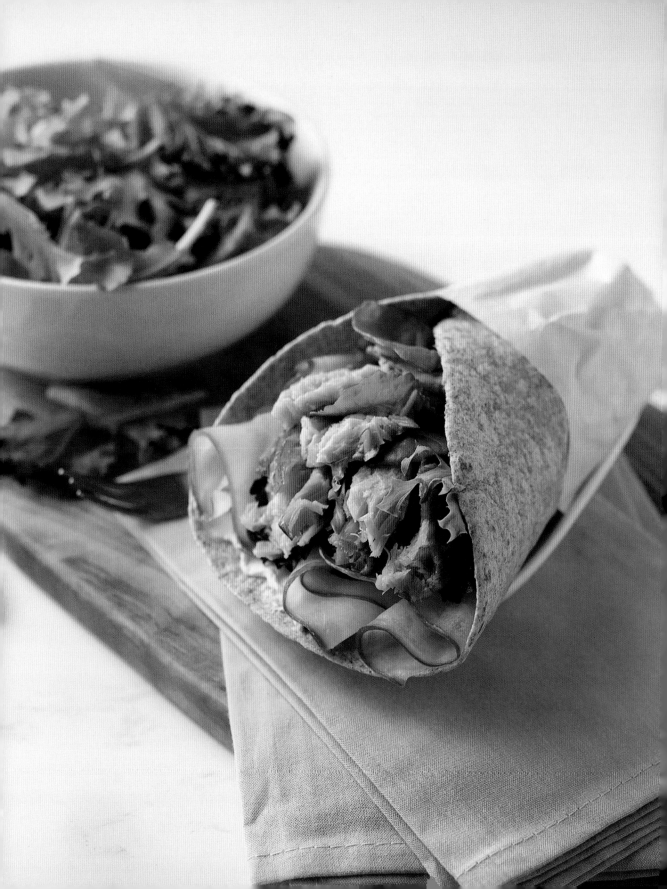

SALMON WRAP WITH VEGGIES AND CREAM CHEESE

■ YIELD:
1 SERVING

■ PREP TIME:
5 MINUTES

■ ASSEMBLY TIME:
5 MINUTES

Here's another wrap that's perfect for a packed lunch. Salmon, an oily fish, is full of omega-3 fatty acids that support both metabolic and brain health, and it's a classic companion for cream cheese. You can use your favorite kind of salmon here: canned, smoked, sushi-grade, a flavored salmon pouch, or even leftover cooked salmon.

⅓ **large cucumber**

2 tablespoons (25 g) whipped cream cheese

1 8-inch (20 cm) Ole Xtreme high-fiber tortilla

4 ounces (115 g) cooked, cured, or sushi grade salmon, such as smoked salmon or canned salmon

Handful of greens, such as spinach, arugula, or lettuce (about 30 g)

Using a Y peeler, slice the cucumber lengthwise to create long thin, thin strips. Set aside.

Spread the cream cheese evenly on the tortilla. Top with the salmon, cucumber strips, and greens. Roll up like an egg roll by folding the bottom over the filling and then rolling in the two sides, and serve.

NOTES

- **Tip:** Don't peel your cucumbers. There's lots of valuable fiber in cucumber peel; it helps stabilize blood sugars.

- **Easy Swap:** If you're not in love with cucumber, load up your wrap with other veggies, such as spinach, lettuce, and/or tomato.

NUTRITIONAL ANALYSIS

SERVING SIZE: 1 wrap

PER SERVING: 294 calories; 13 g fat; 32 g protein; 13 g carbohydrates; 9 g fiber

CHICKEN COWBOY CAVIAR POCKETS

■ **YIELD:**
6 SERVINGS

■ **PREP TIME:**
5 MINUTES

■ **ASSEMBLY TIME:**
5 MINUTES

Don't let the carb count in this recipe scare you. Choosing wholesome, high-fiber carb sources is important for improving insulin sensitivity, and this recipe is jammed with them. Together, beans and corn create a complete protein that your body uses more effectively than the protein contained in one or the other alone. They also have lots of fiber, plus other vitamins and minerals that promote a healthy metabolism.

- 1 (10-ounce/280 g) can shredded chicken, drained and rinsed
- 1 (12-ounce/340 g) can no-sodium-added corn, drained and rinsed
- 1 (15-ounce/400 g) can black beans, drained and rinsed
- 1 (15-ounce/400 g) can no-salt-added black-eyed peas, drained and rinsed
- 1 tomato, diced
- 1 green pepper, diced
- ½ cup (80 g) diced red onion
- 2 tablespoons (1 g) chopped fresh cilantro leaves
- 1½ cups (360 ml) sugar-free Italian dressing
- Black pepper
- 6 whole-grain pita pockets
- 1 large avocado, peeled, pitted, and thinly sliced

Combine the chicken, corn, black beans, black-eyed peas, tomato, green pepper, red onion, cilantro, and Italian dressing in a medium bowl. Mix well and season with black pepper. Refrigerate until you are ready to serve.

To serve, divide the cowboy caviar among the pita pockets and top each with three thin avocado slices. Store the pita pockets at room temperature and the cowboy caviar in the refrigerator for up to 5 days.

NOTES

- **Tips:** This is one of those dishes that's even better the next day. I recommend preparing it ahead of time so that lunch for the week is taken care of. It's also important to note that salad dressings are not labeled as sugar-free, even if they don't contain sugar. To find one, look on the nutrition label for 0 g sugar.

- **Easy Swap:** Eating a variety of beans boosts micronutrients—swap black beans or black-eyed peas as needed. You can use frozen corn instead of canned, heating per package directions first.

NUTRITIONAL ANALYSIS

SERVING SIZE: 1 cup bean and chicken mixture (255 g), 1 pita

PER SERVING: 394 calories; 10 g fat; 27 g protein; 51 g carbohydrates; 10 g fiber

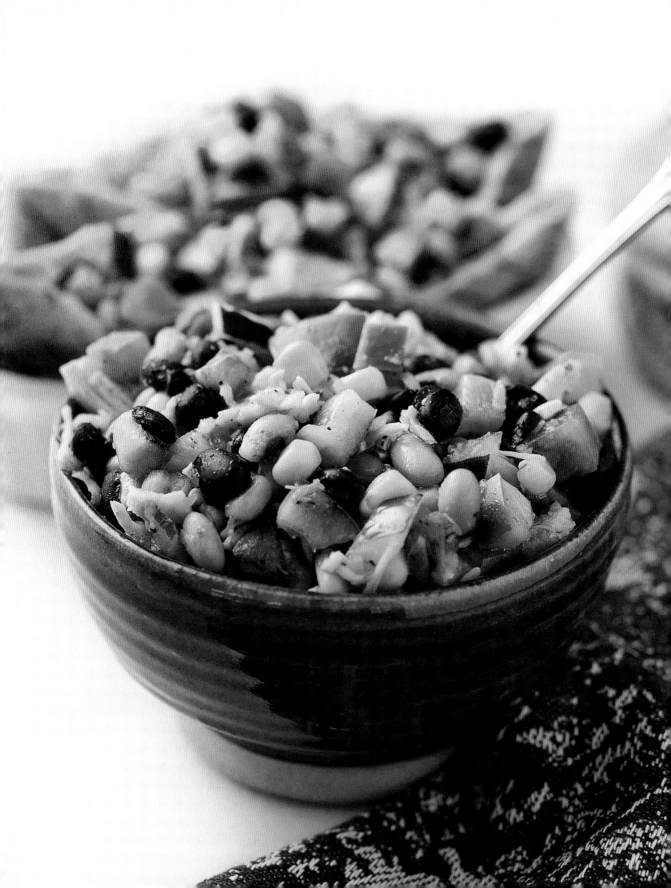

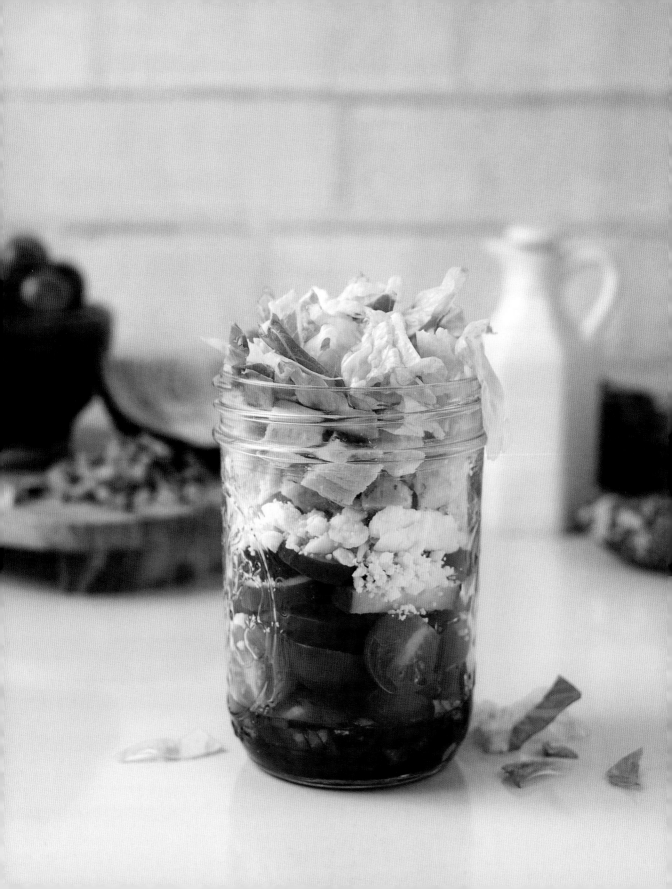

MASON JAR GREEK SALAD

Mason jar salads make packed lunches so much more fun. This one is protein-loaded and full of Mediterranean flavor. Take it to the office (and wait for your coworkers to demand the recipe) or bring it with you on the road you when you're traveling.

■ YIELD:
1 SERVING

■ PREP TIME:
5 MINUTES

■ ASSEMBLY TIME:
5 MINUTES

1 tablespoon (15 ml) olive oil

1 teaspoon balsamic vinegar

Pinch of salt

Pinch of black pepper

1 tablespoon (8 g) chopped red onion

½ cup (80 g) cherry tomatoes, halved

½ cup (75 g) cucumber slices

2 tablespoons (15 g) crumbled feta cheese

4 ounces (115 g) cooked chicken, cubed

1 cup (60 g) chopped romaine lettuce

Whisk together the oil, vinegar, salt, and pepper in a small bowl. Pour into a mason jar. Layer in the remaining ingredients in order: red onion, cherry tomatoes, cucumber, feta, chicken, and lettuce.

Cover tightly, refrigerate, and consume within 3 days. When you are ready to eat, carefully transfer to a plate or shake and eat right from the jar.

NOTES

- **Tip:** If you want to make a batch of these salads for the whole week, go ahead: Just follow the recipe but keep the dressing on the side until you are ready to eat.

- **Easy Swaps:** Replace the chicken with another protein source, like fish, tofu, or beans. Swap out or add any veggies you'd like: I omitted the traditional black olives here because not everyone is a fan, but I think they're a nice touch.

NUTRITIONAL ANALYSIS

SERVING SIZE: 1 jar

PER SERVING: 325 calories; 19 g fat; 31 g protein; 3 g carbohydrates; 3 g fiber

PREP-AHEAD MASON JAR CHICKEN TACO SALAD

■ YIELD:
2 SERVINGS

■ PREP TIME:
10 MINUTES

■ ASSEMBLY TIME:
5 MINUTES

This chicken taco salad is made for volume-eaters, and it's so flavorful that you won't even miss the (high-sodium, processed) tortilla chips. Plus, yogurt-based store-bought dressings tend to be less processed and contain more protein than many others on supermarket shelves.

- 3 tablespoons (45 ml) yogurt-based ranch dressing
- ½ cup (75 g) chopped yellow bell pepper
- ⅔ cup (100 g) halved cherry tomatoes
- 2 ounces (56 g) guacamole, or ½ medium-size avocado, peeled, pitted, and mashed
- ¾ cup (115 g) shredded cooked chicken breast
- ½ cup (80 g) canned black beans, drained and rinsed
- 2 cups (60 g) torn romaine lettuce
- 2 tablespoons (15 g) shredded cheddar cheese
- 2 tablespoons (6 g) sliced green onions, light and dark green parts only (optional)

Add half the dressing to each of two mason jars. To prevent the softer ingredients from getting soggy in the dressing at the bottom, divide and layer the rest of the ingredients into the jars in the following order: bell pepper, cherry tomatoes, guacamole, chicken, black beans, romaine lettuce, cheddar cheese, and green onions.

Cover tightly, refrigerate, and consume within 3 days. When you are ready to eat, carefully transfer to a plate or shake and eat right from the jar.

NOTES

- **Tips:** Prepping lunches for the week ahead of time is essential to staying on track for many people. This is a great example of a high-protein grab-and-go lunch that'll help you avoid a midday stop at a fast-food restaurant.

- **Easy Swaps:** Forgot to precook your chicken breast? Canned chicken works just fine here. Keep some in the pantry for "whoops" moments like these. Alternatively, you can pop some frozen grilled chicken into the microwave and proceed with the recipe.

NUTRITIONAL ANALYSIS

SERVING SIZE: 1 salad

PER SERVING: 230 calories; 9 g fat; 20 g protein; 16 g carbohydrates; 6 g fiber

MIX-AND-MATCH LUNCHBOX

■ **YIELD:**
1 SERVING

■ **ASSEMBLY TIME:**
5 MINUTES

As kids, most of us were taught in school to "eat the rainbow." Well, that was good advice. Consuming a variety of colorful fruits and vegetables is key to getting all the essential vitamins, minerals, and phytonutrients your body needs. That's where this snack-style lunch comes in: It lets you use whatever you have on hand to create a balanced and nourishing midday meal.

PROTEIN (PICK 1):
4 OUNCES (ABOUT 115 G)

Cheese cubes

Cubed chicken breast

Marinated tofu

Lentils

Edamame beans

VEGETABLE (PICK 1 TO 2):
½ CUP EACH (ABOUT 125 G)

Cherry tomatoes

Spinach

Carrots

Celery

Cauliflower

Broccoli

Cucumbers

Pickled beets

FRUIT (PICK 1):
1 CUP (ABOUT 250 G)

Grapes

Apple slices

Orange

Cherries

½ banana

STARCH (PICK 1):
½ CUP (WEIGHT VARIES)

Whole-grain crackers

Corn tortilla chips

Cooked quinoa

Cooked brown rice

Cooked, frozen corn

ADDITIONS (PICK 1):
2 TO 4 TABLESPOONS
(30 TO 60 G)

Nuts

Hummus

Flax or hemp seeds

Choose your favorite options from the lists above (or use your own favorites) and add to a meal prep container or plate. Make sure you get an even mix of ingredients from each category. Enjoy!

NUTRITIONAL ANALYSIS

SERVING SIZE: 1 lunchbox, varies

PER SERVING: varies

NOTES

- **Tips:** Most of the proteins listed are low in fat, but cheese has a high saturated-fat content. This is okay as long as you balance it with low-fat protein options throughout your day. You can always choose to split your protein choice into 2 ounces (40 g) of cheese and 2 ounces of a lean meat (60 g) to meet the 4-ounce goal.

- **Easy Swaps:** There are billions of foods in this world, and this list is incomplete, so add your own favorites to this page and cross out the ones that don't fit your preferences. Just remember that foods that increase insulin sensitivity are high in fiber and protein, and low in added sugar, sodium, and saturated fat.

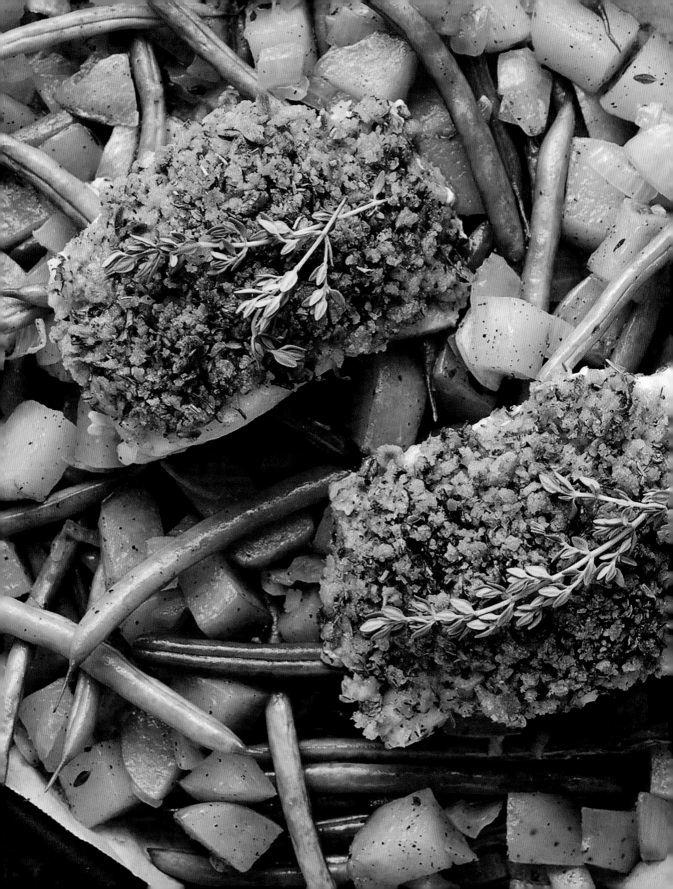

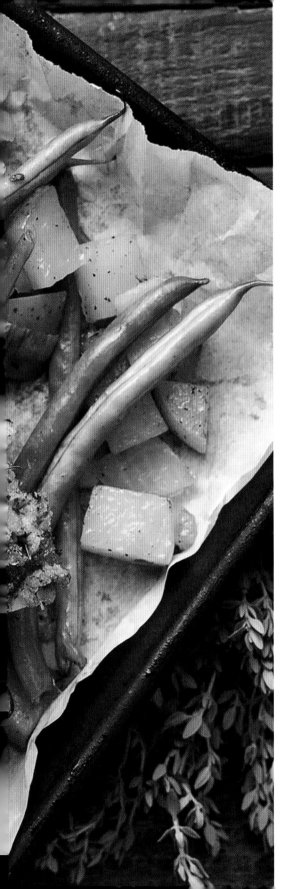

CHAPTER 5

35 Dinners in 35 Minutes

What's the ideal dinner recipe? Well, we all want it to meet three criteria: It should be healthy, something the whole family can enjoy, and it shouldn't mean spending hours in the kitchen. If that sounds like a tall order, keep reading. I'm about to show you that it can be done. The recipes in this chapter prove that an insulin-friendly eating pattern doesn't mean swearing off carbs forever, using obscure or hard-to-find ingredients, or a life sentence of bland and boring food. It means meals that are simple, joyful, colorful, and well-balanced—and great for batch-cooking, too.

CHICKEN PARMESAN WITH BROCCOLI

A healthier version of classic chicken parm, this recipe is just as good as the real thing, with its crisp breaded chicken and lightly chewy pasta. Using chickpea spaghetti is a good way to sneak more protein and fiber into a meal. It's very similar in texture and flavor to regular wheat pastas.

■ **YIELD:**
6 SERVINGS

■ **PREP TIME:**
10 MINUTES

■ **COOK TIME:**
25 MINUTES

3 large chicken breasts

⅓ cup (30 g) whole-wheat dried breadcrumbs

⅓ cup (30 g) grated Parmesan, plus more to serve

3 tablespoons (45 ml) olive oil, divided

16 ounces (450 g) fresh broccoli florets

Salt and black pepper

1 (8.8 ounce/250 g) box chickpea spaghetti

1½ cups (360 ml) no-sugar-added red pasta sauce

1 cup (120 g) low-fat shredded mozzarella cheese

Preheat the oven to 450°F (230°F). Line a 9½ by 13-inch (24 by 33 cm) sheet pan with aluminum foil and lightly coat with cooking spray. Line a second 9½ by 13-inch (24 by 33 cm) sheet pan with parchment paper.

Cut each chicken breast in half horizontally to create thinner fillets.

Combine the breadcrumbs and Parmesan in a shallow bowl. Using a pastry brush, coat both sides of the chicken breasts lightly using 2 tablespoons (30 ml) olive oil total, then dip into the breadcrumb mixture, coating the chicken on all sides. Place each chicken breast on the foil-lined baking sheet, spritz with a little cooking spray, and bake for 15 minutes.

Combine the broccoli florets and 1 tablespoon (15 ml) olive oil in a large mixing bowl and season with salt and pepper. Toss to coat and spread on the parchment-lined baking sheet. Transfer to the oven with the chicken and bake for 20 minutes.

Cook the chickpea spaghetti according to package directions, using the lower end of the recommended cooking time as a guideline. Drain well.

Remove the chicken from the oven and top each chicken fillet with 2 tablespoons (30 ml) of pasta sauce and 2 tablespoons (30 g) of shredded mozzarella cheese. Bake for 5 minutes more, or until the cheese is melted. Turn the broiler to high and broil on the top rack for an additional 2 minutes to brown the cheese.

Divide the pasta evenly among six plates. Top each with about ¼ cup (60 ml) sauce, a chicken breast fillet, and an extra sprinkle of Parmesan, if desired. Store leftovers in an airtight container in the refrigerator up to 5 days.

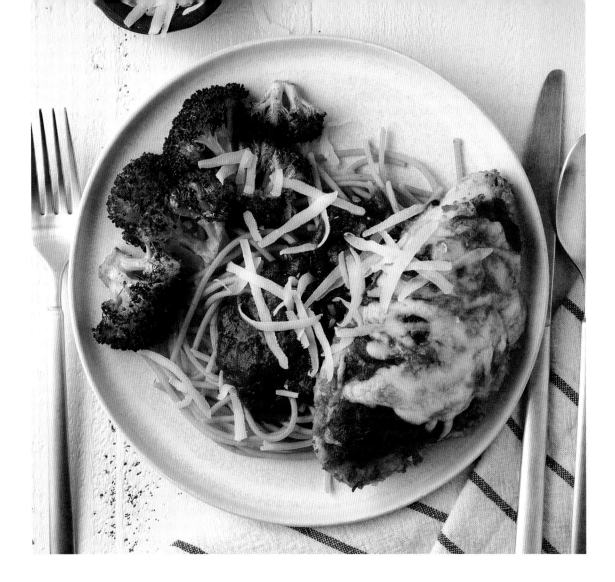

NUTRITIONAL ANALYSIS

SERVING SIZE: 1 cup (200 g) spaghetti, 1 chicken fillet

PER SERVING: 430 calories; 12 g fat; 47 g protein; 38 g carbohydrates; 7 g fiber

NOTES

- **Tip:** Don't skip the step of slicing the chicken breasts in half. It's essential for getting the breaded chicken to become crispy fast.

- **Easy Swaps:** If broccoli doesn't do it for you, swap it with your favorite nonstarchy vegetable, such as cauliflower, carrots. Or replace it with a side salad, such as the simple kale side salad on page 89.

INSULIN-FRIENDLY CARBONARA WITH A SIMPLE KALE SIDE SALAD

■ **YIELD:**
5 SERVINGS

■ **PREP TIME:**
10 MINUTES

■ **COOK TIME:**
20 MINUTES

Traditional carbonara gets a healthy twist here, but never fear—my version is just as rich and creamy. My recipe is higher in fiber and protein and lower in saturated fat than the original. I keep the flavor while reducing the saturated fat content by using less of the rendered bacon fat. The crisp kale side salad adds contrast, color, and crunch.

FOR THE CARBONARA

5 bacon strips, sliced into ¼-inch (6 mm) pieces

1 (8.8-ounce/250 g) package chickpea spaghetti

2 large eggs, at room temperature

2 egg yolks, at room temperature

1 cup (100 g) grated Parmesan cheese, plus more for serving

¼ teaspoon salt

¼ teaspoon black pepper

1 cup (150 g) frozen peas

4 cloves garlic, minced

1 tablespoon (6 g) lemon zest, plus more for serving

Place a skillet over medium heat, add the bacon, and cook until crispy, about 7 minutes, stirring occasionally. Set the bacon aside on a plate lined with a paper towel to absorb extra fat.

Cook the pasta according to package directions. Before draining, reserve ½ cup (120 ml) of the cooking liquid. Drain well.

Meanwhile, whisk the eggs and egg yolks in a large bowl. Gently fold in the Parmesan, salt, and black pepper.

Wipe out the pan in which you cooked the bacon, leaving about 2 tablespoons (30 ml) of bacon fat. Add the peas and cook for 4 minutes. Add the garlic and cook for 1 minute more. Add the bacon, lemon zest, and cooked pasta to the peas and stir until combined.

Add this mixture and ¼ cup (60 ml) of the reserved pasta water to the bowl with the egg mixture, stirring vigorously for 1 minute as the eggs gently cook on the warm pasta, becoming a creamy sauce. If the sauce seems too thick, add more of the remaining pasta water. Divide among five plates and garnish with an extra sprinkle of cheese and lemon zest.

NUTRITIONAL ANALYSIS

SERVING SIZE: 1¾ cups (385 g) carbonara, 1½ cups (40 g) salad

PER SERVING: 521 calories; 31 g fat; 28 g protein; 30 g carbohydrates; 7 g fiber

NOTES

- **Tips:** Don't throw out the two extra egg whites—save them to use in tomorrow's breakfast.

- **Easy Swaps:** If you're feeling fancy, use 5 ounces of pancetta instead of traditional bacon.

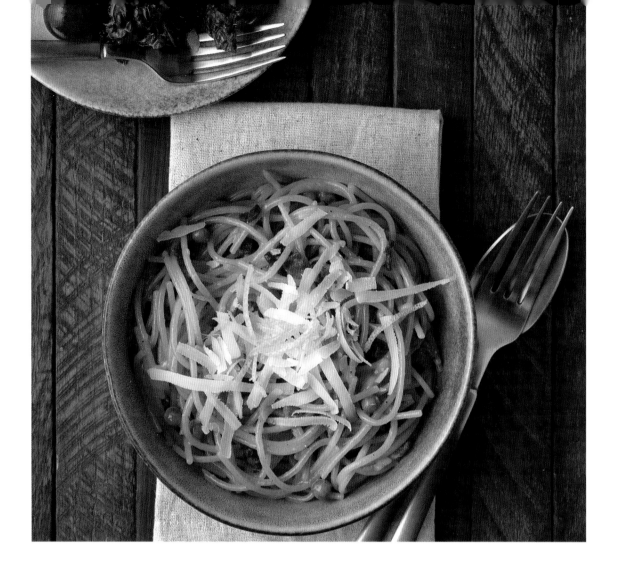

FOR THE KALE SIDE SALAD

4 ounces (115 g) lacinato kale, torn

1 cup (150 g) cherry tomatoes, halved

1 cup (150 g) sliced red onion

¼ cup (60 ml) avocado or olive oil

3 tablespoons (45 ml) red wine vinegar

2 teaspoons (10 g) Dijon mustard

Pinch of garlic salt

To make the kale salad, place the kale, cherry tomatoes, and red onion in a large mixing bowl. Add the oil, vinegar, mustard, and garlic salt to a jar and shake well. Pour over the vegetables and toss until combined. Divide among five bowls and serve with the pasta. Since kale, tomato, and onion are hardy vegetables, this kale salad will stay fresh in the refrigerator for up to 3 days.

CREAMY SPINACH STUFFED CHICKEN WITH SWEET POTATOES

■ **YIELD:**
4 SERVINGS

■ **PREP TIME:**
10 MINUTES

■ **COOK TIME:**
30 MINUTES

If you're starving and need a hearty meal, this one's for you. Juicy chicken stuffed with creamy spinach and roasted sweet potatoes make a balanced, satisfying dinner that keeps you full for hours.

4 large boneless, skinless chicken breasts

½ teaspoon paprika

½ teaspoon chili powder

¾ teaspoon salt

½ teaspoon garlic powder

½ teaspoon onion powder

¼ cup (45 g) whipped cream cheese

⅓ cup (85 g) plain nonfat Greek yogurt

⅓ cup (40 g) grated Parmesan cheese

1½ cups (45 g) chopped fresh spinach

½ teaspoon dried red pepper flakes

2 medium-size sweet potatoes

1 tablespoon (15 ml) olive oil

⅛ teaspoon black pepper

Preheat the oven to 375°F (190°C). Line a 9½ by 13-inch (24 by 33 cm) sheet pan with parchment paper. Coat a 9 by 13-inch (23 by 33 cm) baking dish with cooking spray.

Cut each chicken breast horizontally three-quarters of the way through to create a space for stuffing.

In a small bowl, combine the paprika, chili powder, ½ teaspoon of the salt, garlic powder, and onion powder. Rub evenly over both sides of each chicken breast.

In a large mixing bowl, combine the cream cheese, Greek yogurt, Parmesan, spinach, and red pepper flakes. Stuff one-quarter of this mixture into each chicken breast. Place in a single layer on the parchment covered sheet pan and bake for 30 minutes.

Meanwhile, peel and cube the sweet potatoes into ¾-inch (2 cm) pieces. Toss with the olive oil, the remaining ¼ teaspoon salt, and black pepper in a separate large mixing bowl. Transfer to the prepared baking dish and roast for 25 minutes.

When done, let the chicken cool for 5 minutes before serving with the roasted sweet potatoes.

NUTRITIONAL ANALYSIS

SERVING SIZE: 1 stuffed chicken breast, ½ cup (100 g) sweet potatoes

PER SERVING: 366 calories; 10 g fat; 47 g protein; 22 g carbohydrates; 4 g fiber

NOTES

- **Tip:** Let the cream cheese warm to room temperature before using; It'll take less elbow grease to mix.

- **Easy Swaps:** You can swap Greek yogurt with cottage cheese for a similarly creamy texture. Butternut squash is a good seasonal swap for sweet potatoes.

SHEET-PAN PORK CHOPS WITH BABY POTATOES AND ASPARAGUS

Another one-pan dinner solution. Tender marinated pork chops, crisp asparagus, and golden baby potatoes combine for a wholesome meal with plenty of fiber and protein and minimal cleanup.

YIELD:
4 SERVINGS

PREP TIME:
10 MINUTES

COOK TIME:
30 MINUTES

1 pound (450 g) baby potatoes, quartered

1 tablespoon plus 1 teaspoon (20 ml) olive oil

Salt and black pepper

¼ cup (60 ml) low-sodium soy sauce

2 tablespoons (24 g) brown sugar alternative

2 teaspoons (10 ml) Worcestershire sauce

1 teaspoon Dijon mustard

1½ teaspoons apple cider vinegar

2 teaspoons (6 g) minced garlic

½ teaspoon chili powder

4 lean boneless pork chops, about 5 ounces (140 g) each or 1¼ pounds (560 g) total

1 pound (450 g) asparagus spears, woody ends removed

Preheat the oven to 400°F (200°C). Line an 18 by 26-inch (45 by 66 cm) sheet pan with parchment paper.

Toss the potatoes with 1 tablespoon (15 ml) of the olive oil and a pinch each of salt and pepper. Spread evenly on the sheet pan and roast for 10 minutes.

Meanwhile, whisk together the soy sauce, brown sugar alternative, Worcestershire sauce, mustard, vinegar, garlic, chili powder, and ⅛ teaspoon black pepper in a shallow bowl. Place the pork chops in the bowl, coat with the marinade, and set aside.

Toss the asparagus spears with the remaining 1 teaspoon olive oil and a pinch of salt and pepper. When the roasting time for the potatoes is up, remove the pan from the oven and push the potatoes over to one half of the pan. Add the asparagus in a single layer to the other half. Return to the oven for 5 minutes.

Remove the pan from the oven and push the veggies to one side. Add the pork chops (discarding any excess marinade) and bake for another 15 minutes, until they reach an internal temperature of 145°F (63°C). Turn the broiler to high and broil on the top rack for an additional 2 to 3 minutes for a caramelized top on the pork chops.

Serve immediately.

NUTRITIONAL ANALYSIS

SERVING SIZE: 4-ounce (115 g) pork chop, ½ cup (125 g) baby potatoes, about 6 asparagus spears

PER SERVING: 513 calories; 30 g fat; 29 g protein; 25 g carbohydrates; 5 g fiber

NOTES

- **Tip:** If you don't have a shallow bowl, marinating the pork chops in a resealable plastic bag also works well.

- **Easy Swaps:** Substitute chicken breasts for pork, if you prefer. Green beans work well in place of asparagus.

CREAMY MUSHROOM CHICKEN WITH TOMATOES AND SPINACH

■ YIELD:
4 SERVINGS

■ PREP TIME:
5 MINUTES

■ COOK TIME:
25 MINUTES

You'll want to put this creamy chicken dish on your repeat list. The sauce has "cold winter's evening" written all over it, and it's got lots of colorful vegetables and protein for balance. This recipe contains about 8 grams of saturated fat per serving, falling well within the daily guideline of 25 grams, but it might be a good idea to make it on a day when you're not planning to consume other foods high in saturated fats (like fried foods or a rich dessert).

1½ cups (280 g) uncooked basmati rice

2 large boneless, skinless chicken breasts

Salt and black pepper

2 tablespoons (30 ml) olive oil

3 tablespoons (45 g) unsalted butter

2 cups (300 g) cherry tomatoes

4 garlic cloves, minced

2 cups (150 g) sliced mushrooms

5 ounces (140 g) fresh spinach

¾ cup (180 ml) low-sodium chicken broth

1 teaspoon lemon juice

½ teaspoon salt

½ teaspoon garlic powder

1 cup (240 ml) whole milk

Chopped fresh parsley, for garnish

Cook the rice according to package directions or use a rice cooker.

Meanwhile, cut the chicken breasts in halves horizontally to create four thinner cutlets. Season with salt and pepper.

Add 1 tablespoon (15 ml) olive oil and 1 tablespoon (15 g) butter to a high-sided skillet over medium-high heat. Once the pan is hot, add the chicken and cook for 4 minutes on each side, or until they reach an internal temperature of 165°F (75°C). Remove the cooked chicken and set aside.

Meanwhile, heat 1 tablespoon (15 ml) olive oil in a separate large skillet over medium-high heat. Add the cherry tomatoes and cook until blistered, stirring occasionally, about 6 minutes.

Place the skillet in which you cooked the chicken over medium heat. Melt the remaining 2 tablespoons (30 g) butter. Add the garlic and mushrooms and saute for 7 minutes or until mushrooms are softened. Add the spinach and cook, covered, until wilted, about 2 minutes.

Add the cooked cherry tomatoes, chicken broth, lemon juice, salt, and garlic powder to the skillet. Let it cook, uncovered, for 5 minutes, or until the liquid is reduced by about a third.

Stir in the milk, return the chicken to the pan, and cook for another 5 minutes, stirring frequently, until texture of the sauce is creamy and slightly thickened.

Divide the cooked rice among four plates, top each with equal portions of chicken, veggies, and sauce, and garnish with the parsley.

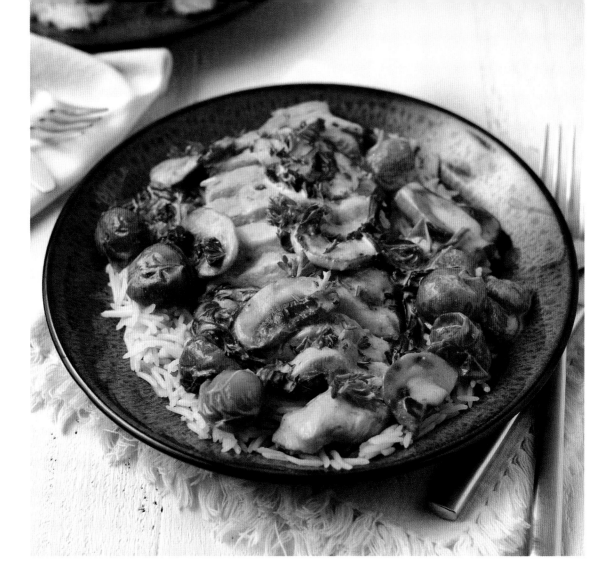

NUTRITIONAL ANALYSIS

SERVING SIZE: 1 chicken cutlet,
¾ cup (150 g) cooked rice, 1 cup
(250 g) veggies and sauce

PER SERVING: 528 calories;
20 g fat; 41 g protein;
46 g carbohydrates; 4 g fiber

NOTES

- **Tip:** To make this a one-pot meal, don't blister the tomatoes: Cut them in half and add them with the mushrooms instead. This doesn't really save time, but it does mean you'll have one less dirty pan when you're done.

- **Easy Swap:** Use eight boneless, skinless chicken thighs instead of four breasts.

CHICKEN SAUSAGE SIZZLE BOWL

Grain bowls are all the rage these days, and I love this one—it's simple but flavorful, with a beautiful color palette. Thanks to the cauliflower rice base, it's also relatively moderate in carbs. And yes, sausage is a processed meat, but enjoying it in moderation can be part of a healthy eating pattern. I believe in a sustainable approach that promotes overall health and well-being without being overly restrictive.

■ **YIELD:**
4 SERVINGS

■ **PREP TIME:**
10 MINUTES

■ **COOK TIME:**
20 MINUTES

■ **ASSEMBLY TIME:**
5 MINUTES

2 small sweet potatoes

12 ounces (340 g) brussels sprouts

1 tablespoon (15 ml) olive oil

1 teaspoon Old Bay seasoning

1 pound (450 g) chicken apple sausage

1 tablespoon (15 ml) toasted sesame oil

12 ounces (340 g) frozen cauliflower rice

2 tablespoons (30 ml) beef broth

½ teaspoon salt

Balsamic vinegar or hot sauce (optional)

Preheat the oven to 400°F (200°C). Line a 9½ by 13-inch (24 by 33 cm) sheet pan with parchment paper.

Peel and cut the sweet potatoes into ¾-inch (2 cm) chunks. Trim and halve the brussels sprouts. Toss both with the olive oil and Old Bay seasoning. Spread out on the prepared sheet pan and roast for 20 minutes. Set aside.

Meanwhile, cut the chicken sausages in half lengthwise, then slice into bite-size chunks. Saute in a large skillet over medium-high heat until browned, about 10 minutes.

In a separate skillet, heat the sesame oil over medium heat. Add the cauliflower rice, beef broth, and salt. Stir to combine and cook for 3 to 5 minutes, until the liquid has evaporated, stirring frequently.

Divide the cauliflower rice, chicken sausage, and veggies equally among four bowls. Drizzle with balsamic vinegar or your favorite hot sauce, if using.

NOTES

- **Tips:** This is an especially easy dish to double, so it's great if you're cooking for a large group or doing meal prep for the whole family. You can store it in the refrigerator for up to 6 days.

- **Easy Swaps:** The sweet potatoes add a moderate amount of carbohydrate to this dish, but if you need more, swap the cauliflower rice for jasmine or basmati rice. Wild rice is even better, with triple the fiber of other rice varieties.

NUTRITIONAL ANALYSIS

SERVING SIZE: 1 chicken sausage link, 2 cups (300 g) veggies

PER SERVING: 330 calories; 12 g fat; 18 g protein; 36 g carbohydrates; 8 g fiber

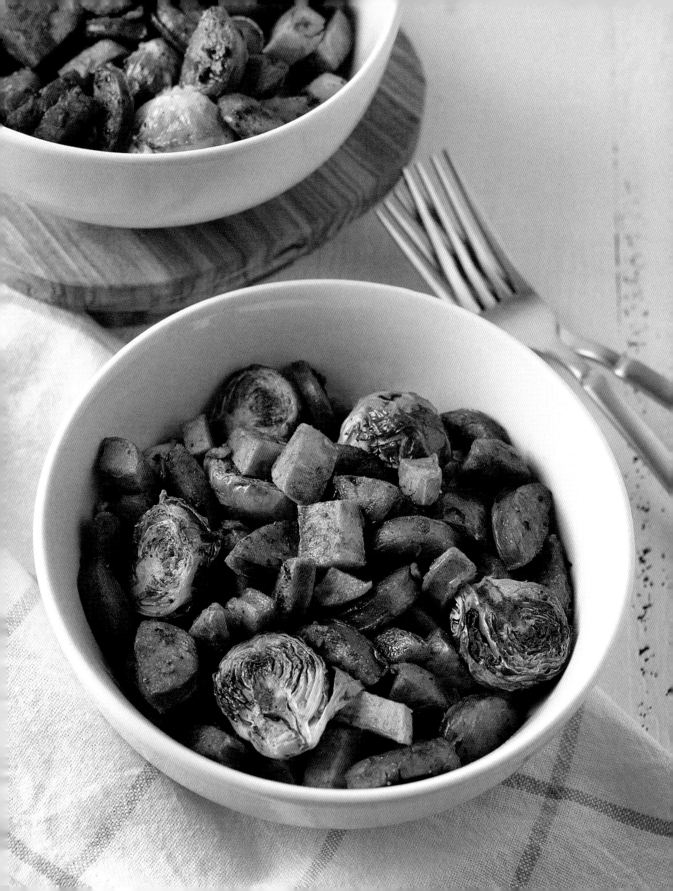

SPAGHETTI SQUASH WITH MEAT SAUCE AND ASPARAGUS

■ YIELD:
4 SERVINGS

■ PREP TIME:
20 MINUTES

■ COOK TIME:
60 MINUTES

Spaghetti squash is a fiber-rich, low-carb pasta swap perfect for balanced meals. This dish combines roasted squash, savory meat sauce, and asparagus for a hearty, nutritious dinner.

2 medium-size spaghetti squash

3 tablespoons (45 ml) olive oil

1 teaspoon salt, plus more as needed

Black pepper

1 pound (450 g) lean ground beef

2 shallots, chopped

1 large carrot, grated

1 pound (450 g) asparagus spears, woody ends trimmed

¼ cup (60 ml) dry red wine

¼ cup (60 g) tomato paste

½ cup (120 ml) water

2 cloves garlic, minced

1 teaspoon dried oregano

1 teaspoon dried parsley

1 cup (240 g) ricotta cheese

2 cups (200 g) shredded low-fat mozzarella cheese

Grated Parmesan cheese (optional)

Preheat the oven to 425°F (220°C). Line a 9½ by 13-inch (24 by 33 cm) sheet pan with parchment paper.

Cut each spaghetti squash in half lengthwise and scoop out the seeds. Drizzle lightly with 2 tablespoons (30 ml) of the olive oil and season with pinches of salt and pepper. Place cut side down on the baking sheet and bake for 60 minutes, or until the shell of the squash gives when you push on it.

In the last 15 minutes of baking, heat a large skillet over medium heat. Add the ground beef, shallots, and carrots, and brown for about 6 minutes.

Place a separate skillet with the remaining 1 tablespoon (15 ml) olive oil over medium heat. Add the asparagus and sprinkle with salt and pepper. Cook, turning occasionally, for about 6 minutes, until the asparagus is crisp-tender.

Once the meat is browned, add the red wine and stir until evaporated. Add the tomato paste, water, garlic, oregano, parsley, and 1 teaspoon salt. Stir well and saute for about 2 minutes more, until the mixture is heated thoroughly.

When the spaghetti squash are done, flip over and gently pull the flesh from the rind using two forks. It should form noodle-like strands. Drop ¼ cup (65 g) ricotta into each squash half, top with one-quarter of the meat sauce, then sprinkle with ½ cup (110 g) mozzarella. Return the squash halves to the oven, turn the broiler to high, and broil on the top rack for 2 to 3 minutes, until the mozzarella is melted and lightly browned. Top with grated Parmesan cheese, if desired, and serve alongside the asparagus spears.

NUTRITIONAL ANALYSIS

SERVING SIZE: ½ spaghetti squash

PER SERVING: 570 calories; 32 g fat; 27 g protein; 49 g carbohydrates; 11 g fiber

SLOW-COOKER TURKEY MEATBALL SOUP

■ YIELD:
6 SERVINGS

■ PREP TIME:
15 MINUTES

■ COOK TIME:
3 TO 7 HOURS

Traditional meatball soup is high in saturated fat, so I've lightened it up with less fat and added beans for fiber and protein. This insulin-friendly version is easy with a slow cooker—just prep in the morning, and dinner's ready when you get home.

1 medium-size yellow onion, chopped

1 large carrot, chopped

1 celery stalk, chopped

12 ounces (340 g) frozen cut green beans

1 medium-size zucchini, chopped

1½ cups (240 g) great northern beans, drained and rinsed

2 tablespoons (18 g) minced garlic

2 teaspoons (1.5 g) dried parsley

2 teaspoons (1.5 g) dried oregano

2 teaspoons (1.5 g) dried basil

2 bay leaves

1 teaspoon salt

½ teaspoon black pepper

3 tablespoons (45 ml) lemon juice

20 ounces (570 g) turkey meatballs

1 (14-ounce/400 g) can diced tomatoes

5 cups (1.2 L) low-sodium chicken or vegetable broth

Combine the onion, carrot, celery, green beans, zucchini, great northern beans, garlic, parsley, oregano, basil, bay leaves, salt, black pepper, lemon juice, meatballs, tomatoes, and broth in a slow cooker. Stir to combine. Cook on high for 3 to 4 hours, or low for 6 to 7 hours. Remove the bay leaves before serving.

NUTRITIONAL ANALYSIS

SERVING SIZE: 2 cups (475 ml)

PER SERVING: 296 calories; 10 g fat; 27 g protein; 23 g carbohydrates; 6 g fiber

NOTES

- **Tips:** It does mean an extra step, but sautéing the onion, carrot, and celery in 1 tablespoon (15 ml) of olive oil before adding it to the slow-cooker will give the soup a richer flavor.

- **Easy Swaps:** I prefer chicken broth for its deeper flavor, even in vegetable soups, but if you'd like to make this soup vegan, you can substitute vegetable broth and meat-alternative meatballs or cubed firm tofu.

SLOW-COOKER BRAISED ROAST WITH ROOT VEGETABLES

YIELD:
6 SERVINGS

PREP TIME:
30 MINUTES

COOK TIME:
4 TO 8 HOURS

Slow-cooker meals are lifesavers when you have a busy day ahead because you can throw the ingredients into the slow cooker in the morning and then let it do all the work for you. This one is rich, savory, and comforting, and uses low-carb (and highly underrated) turnips in place of potatoes (not that potatoes can't be a part of an insulin-friendly eating pattern, of course).

---

2 teaspoons (4 g) ground cinnamon

½ teaspoon ground allspice

½ teaspoon cayenne pepper

2 teaspoons (10 g) salt

½ teaspoon black pepper

2½ to 3 pounds (1.1 to 1.4 kg) chuck roast

2 tablespoons (30 ml) avocado oil

1 medium-size onion

3 cloves garlic

5 medium-size carrots

2 large or 3 medium-size turnips

1 cup (240 ml) dry red wine

1 (28-ounce can/800 g) can San Marzano tomatoes

Combine the cinnamon, allspice, cayenne, salt, and pepper in a small bowl. Rub into the roast on all sides.

Heat the avocado oil in a skillet over medium-high heat. Place the roast in the skillet and lightly brown for about 3 minutes per side.

Meanwhile, slice the onion, mince the garlic, and cut carrots and turnips into 1-inch (2.5 cm) chunks.

Remove the roast from the skillet and place into a 6- to 8-quart (5.7 to 7.5 L) slow cooker.

Add the onions and garlic to the skillet and saute for 2 minutes, until the onions soften and turn transparent. Add the wine and cook for 1 minute, scraping any brown bits off the bottom with a wooden spoon. Add the tomatoes and continue scraping as you as break up the tomatoes with your spoon, cooking for 1 minute more.

Add the carrots and turnips to the sauce mixture, then combine until the vegetables are lightly covered with sauce. Pour everything over the roast in the slow cooker.

Slow cook for 4 hours on high or 8 hours on low. When done, slice the roast and serve alongside the root vegetables.

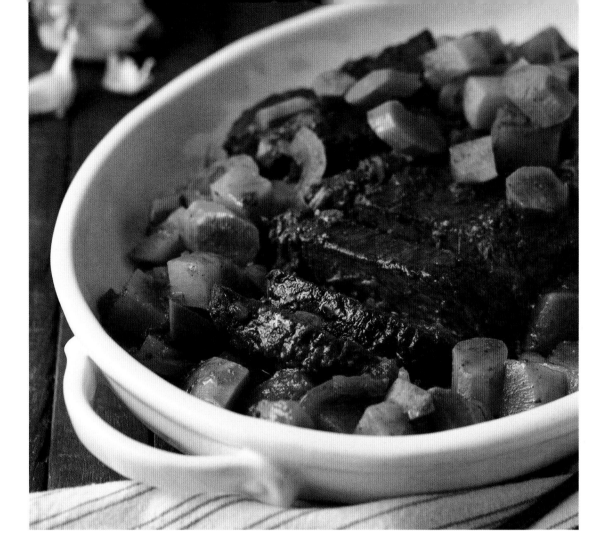

NOTES

- **Tips:** Using an Instant Pot allows you to sauté and cook in one pot so there's less cleaning up to do. If you're using one, you can choose the slow-cook option or cook quickly under pressure.

- **Easy Swaps:** Use crushed tomatoes in place of whole. If you do not have red wine, balsamic vinegar will do the trick. You can also use chicken breasts or pork roast instead of beef, if you prefer. To ensure the same cooking time, use the same weight called for in the ingredients list.

NUTRITIONAL ANALYSIS

SERVING SIZE: 4 ounces (113 g) roast, 1½ cups (250 g) veggies

PER SERVING: 445 calories; 18 g fat; 48 g protein; 14 g carbohydrates; 4 g fiber

HOMEMADE PIZZA, 3 WAYS

My three-ingredient crust is fluffy, chewy, and crispy, with Greek yogurt for protein and calcium, and whole-grain flour for fiber. Together, they lower the glycemic effect of the crust. Which variation will be your new favorite?

YIELD:
1 PIZZA

PREP TIME:
10 MINUTES

COOK TIME:
15 MINUTES

FOR THE CRUST

1⅓ cups (160 g) whole-wheat flour

1 cup (240 g) nonfat plain Greek yogurt

2 teaspoons (8 g) baking powder

PESTO MOZZARELLA

½ cup (120 ml) pesto sauce (fresh pesto, if possible)

6 ounces (170 g) sliced low-fat mozzarella

ROASTED GARLIC

½ cup (120 ml) no-sugar-added red pasta sauce

Handful of fresh spinach

½ cup (120 g) ricotta

4 ounces (115 g) sliced low-fat mozzarella

8 to 12 cloves roasted garlic

Sliced jalapeño (optional)

SUPER CHEESY

½ cup (120 ml) no-sugar-added red pasta sauce

6 ounces (170 g) sliced low-fat mozzarella

½ cup (120 g) ricotta cheese

NUTRITIONAL ANALYSIS (Pesto Mozzarella version)

SERVING SIZE: ⅓ pizza

PER SERVING: 586 calories; 32 g fat; 29 g protein; 46 g carbohydrates; 8 g fiber

Preheat the oven to 425°F (220°C). Line a 9½ by 13-inch (24 by 33 cm) sheet pan with parchment paper and dust lightly with 1 tablespoon (7 g) of flour.

To make the crust, combine the flour, yogurt, and baking powder in a large mixing bowl. Mix well with a rubber spatula until it forms a ball of dough. Using your hands, incorporate all the remaining flour in the bowl into the dough. Knead just enough to make sure it is well combined.

Using your hands and a rolling pin, spread the dough on the baking sheet until about ⅓ inch (8 mm) thick. Spread with sauce, then add the toppings.

Bake for 10 to 12 minutes or until the cheese is melty and the crust is slightly browned. Then turn the broiler on high and broil on the top rack for an additional 1 to 2 minutes, until the cheese is lightly browned.

NOTES

- **Tips:** Add your favorite pizza spice blend to any of the above: It really elevates the flavor of any homemade pizza.

- **Easy Swaps:** When it comes to toppings, the world is your oyster. Choose nongreasy, low- to moderate-fat proteins, and make sure to add at least one veggie for additional fiber.

CORN CREMA CHICKEN ON SPRING GREENS

■ YIELD:
4 SERVINGS

■ PREP TIME:
10 MINUTES

■ COOK TIME:
5 MINUTES

Inspired by Mexican street corn, or elotes, this salad takes only a few minutes to prepare, so it's just the thing if you need a quick on-the-go meal. Cotija cheese adds a nice, salty finish; keep this in mind when you're adding seasoning to the veggie mixture.

- 1 (10-ounce/280 g) bag frozen corn
- 1 (10-ounce/280 g) can chicken breast, drained
- ¼ cup (40 g) diced radishes
- ¼ cup (40 g) coarsely chopped green onions, light and dark green parts only
- 1 tablespoon (15 ml) lime juice
- ⅓ cup (80 g) chipotle mayonnaise
- Salt and black pepper
- 8 cups (240 g) spring greens
- ¼ cup (30 g) crumbled cotija cheese
- ¼ teaspoon chili powder

Place an empty metal bowl in the freezer; you will use it to cool the corn after cooking.

Place the frozen corn in a dry medium-size skillet over medium-high heat. Cook for about 10 minutes, until browned and popping.

Meanwhile, combine the chicken, radishes, and green onions in a large mixing bowl, followed by the lime juice, chipotle mayo, and salt and pepper. Mix well.

Cool the cooked corn by tossing it into the chilled metal bowl and letting it rest for a couple minutes. (The corn doesn't need to cool completely before it's added to the chicken mixture; it just needs to be warm rather than hot, so it doesn't wilt the green onion and warm the mayo.) Mix the corn into the chicken mixture.

When you are ready to serve, divide the greens among four bowls. Top with equal portions of corn chicken salad and cotija cheese and a sprinkle of chili powder.

NUTRITIONAL ANALYSIS

SERVING SIZE: ¾ cup (105 g) corn mixture, 2 cups (35 g) greens, 1 tablespoon (5 g) cotija

PER SERVING: 298 calories; 12 g fat; 23 g protein; 23 g carbohydrates; 3 g fiber

NOTES

- **Tips:** This dish is delicious over a bed of greens, but it's also great as a side dish or appetizer, without the greens. Try serving it as a dip with crackers.

- **Easy Swap:** Replace the green onion with chopped red onion.

ROASTED SUMMER SQUASH AND ARUGULA SALAD WITH MARINATED PORK LOIN

■ YIELD:
4 SERVINGS

■ PREP TIME:
10 MINUTES

■ COOK TIME:
30 MINUTES

■ ASSEMBLY TIME:
5 MINUTES

Raw and roasted veggies work together in this low-carb salad, varying the textures without creating a lot of extra work. Add a side of quinoa or couscous if you need more carbohydrates with your meal.

FOR THE PORK LOIN

- ¼ cup (60 ml) olive oil
- 2 tablespoons (30 ml) low-sodium soy sauce or coconut aminos
- 2 tablespoons (42 g) honey
- 1 tablespoon (15 ml) red wine vinegar
- 1 tablespoon (15 ml) lemon juice
- 1 teaspoon Worcestershire sauce
- 1 teaspoon Dijon mustard
- 1 teaspoon minced garlic
- 2 teaspoons (1.5 g) dried parsley
- ¼ teaspoon black pepper
- 16 ounces (450 g) pork loin

To prepare the pork loin, make a marinade by combining the olive oil, soy sauce or coconut aminos, honey, vinegar, lemon juice, Worcestershire sauce, Dijon mustard, garlic, parsley, and pepper in a small bowl. Whisk together. Transfer to a resealable plastic bag and add the pork loin. Ideally, marinate for at least 4 hours or up to 1 day.

Preheat the oven to 400°F (200°C). Line two 9½ by 13-inch (24 by 33 cm) sheet pans with parchment paper.

Place the pork roast on one sheet pan (discarding any excess marinade) and roast for 30 minutes, flipping halfway through. When done, let the pork rest for 5 minutes.

NUTRITIONAL ANALYSIS

ERVING SIZE: 4 ounces (113 g) pork loin, 3 cups (300 g) salad

PER SERVING: 438 calories; 26 g fat: 24 g protein; 24 g carbohydrates; 7 g fiber

NOTES

- **Tips:** Don't be afraid of adding a little sweetness to your marinades. The meat won't absorb it all, so you'll get tender meat and a touch of sweetness with negligible added sugar per serving. The dressing is the same as the one in the Cherry Tomato and White Bean Salad with White Fish on page 107; it'll jazz up just about any salad.

- **Easy Swap:** If you don't eat pork, chicken breasts or thighs will work well here. Adjust the cooking time as necessary.

FOR THE ROASTED VEGETABLES

1 zucchini, halved and thinly sliced

1 summer squash, halved and thinly sliced

1 tablespoon (15 ml) olive oil

¼ teaspoon salt

⅛ teaspoon black pepper

FOR THE DRESSING

¼ cup (60 ml) olive oil

3 tablespoons (45 ml) red wine vinegar

½ teaspoon salt

½ teaspoon Dijon mustard

½ teaspoon black pepper

2 cloves garlic, minced

1 medium-size shallot, thinly sliced

TO ASSEMBLE

8 cups (240 g) arugula

8 dates, pitted and chopped

To prepare the roasted vegetables, toss the zucchini and summer squash with the oil, salt, and pepper. Spread out evenly on the second sheet pan and roast for 25 minutes.

To make the dressing, combine the olive oil, vinegar, salt, mustard, pepper, garlic, and shallot in a small bowl or jar. Whisk or shake to blend well.

To assemble, put one-quarter of the arugula on each of four plates. Top each with ¾ cup (125 g) roasted veggies, 2 chopped dates, and 2 tablespoons (30 ml) of dressing, making sure to include some shallots. Slice the pork loin and serve on the side.

HIGH-PROTEIN FETA PASTA BAKE

This is my insulin-friendly spin on a viral feta pasta bake. Mine is higher in protein and fiber and more moderate in carbohydrates, since it's loaded with veggies and uses less pasta. Insulin resistance doesn't mean you have to say goodbye to pasta forever.

■ **YIELD:**
5 SERVINGS

■ **PREP TIME:**
10 MINUTES

■ **COOK TIME:**
45 MINUTES

1 (11-ounce/310 g) block feta cheese

2 large boneless, skinless chicken breasts, sliced into 1-inch pieces

2 teaspoons (4 g) onion powder

2 teaspoons (4 g) garlic powder

½ teaspoon salt

½ teaspoon black pepper

3 cloves garlic, minced

Dried red pepper flakes

2 cups (300 g) cherry tomatoes

2 cups (200 g) chopped cauliflower

3 tablespoons (45 ml) olive oil

2 cups (150 g) dry whole-wheat rotini pasta

Preheat the oven to 400°F (200°C.) Coat a 9 by 13-inch (23 by 33 cm) baking dish with cooking spray.

Drain the liquid from the feta and place the whole slab in the center of the pan. Add the chicken in a single layer around the feta (without covering it).

Sprinkle the chicken and feta all over with the onion powder, garlic powder, salt, black pepper, garlic, and red pepper flakes. Spread the cherry tomatoes and cauliflower evenly around the chicken and feta. Drizzle with the olive oil.

Bake for 35 to 40 minutes, until the chicken is cooked through.

Meanwhile, cook the pasta according to package directions. Drain well.

When the chicken and veggies are ready, stir everything together carefully, breaking up the slab of feta, to create a sauce with the feta and juices released during cooking. Add the pasta and stir to combine.

Let rest for 5 minutes, stir again, and serve. Store leftovers in an airtight container in the refrigerator for up to 4 days.

NOTES

- **Tips:** Make sure to cut the chicken into bite-size pieces so that they cook evenly and thoroughly.

- **Easy Swaps:** Swap out cauliflower for coarsely chopped turnips, parsnips, or even broccoli. Use chickpea pasta in place of whole-grain to add even more protein and fiber.

NUTRITIONAL ANALYSIS

SERVING SIZE: 2 cups (300 g)

PER SERVING: 463 calories; 23 g fat; 37 g protein; 29 g carbohydrates; 3 g fiber

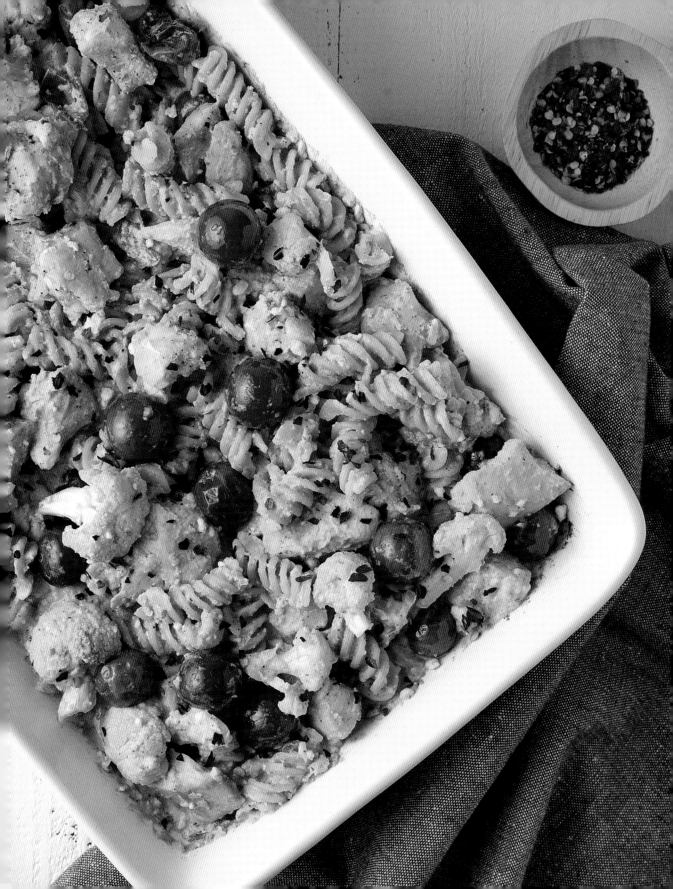

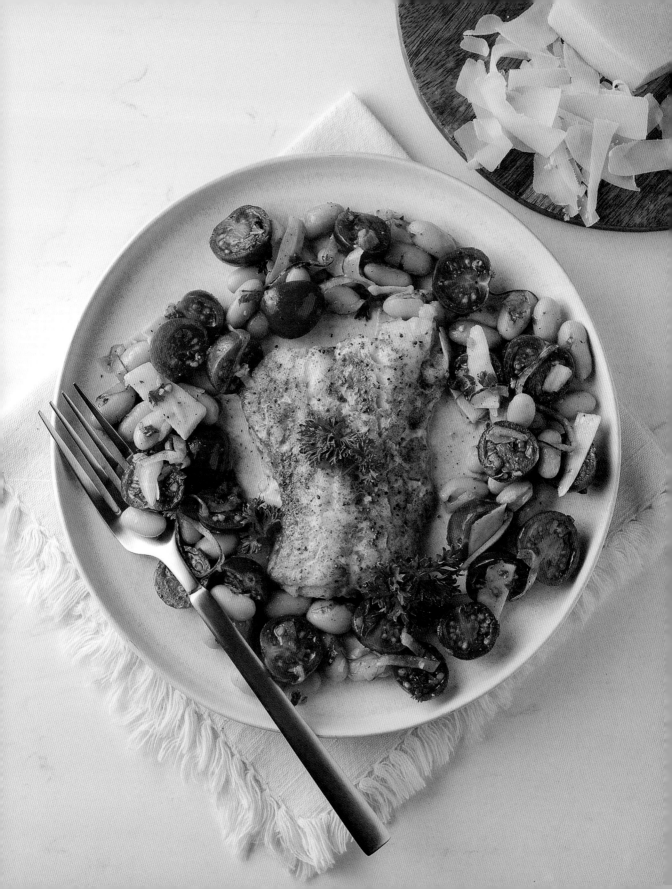

CHERRY TOMATO AND WHITE BEAN SALAD WITH WHITE FISH

YIELD:
4 SERVINGS

PREP TIME:
10 MINUTES

COOK TIME:
15 MINUTES

This vibrant meal pairs a bright tomato, parsley, and bean salad with your favorite mild white fish for a light dinner (or lunch) that's ideal for slightly-more-sedentary days when you're not running around and don't require quite as much energy from your food.

- ¼ cup plus 1 tablespoon (75 ml) olive oil
- 3 tablespoons (45 ml) red wine vinegar
- ½ teaspoon salt
- ½ teaspoon Dijon mustard
- ½ teaspoon black pepper
- 2 cloves garlic, minced
- ½ cup (50 g) thinly sliced red onion
- 24 ounces (680 g) white fish, such as halibut or cod
- 1 tablespoon (15 ml) olive oil
- 2 teaspoons (4 g) Old Bay seasoning
- 4 cups (600 g) cherry tomatoes, halved
- 1 (15-ounce/400 g) can cannellini beans, rinsed and drained
- ¼ cup (10 g) chopped fresh parsley
- ½ cup (50 g) shaved Parmesan cheese

Preheat the oven to 400°F (200°C). Line a 9½ by 13-inch (24 by 33 cm) sheet pan with parchment paper.

In a large bowl, whisk together the ¼ cup (60 ml) of the olive oil, vinegar, salt, mustard, pepper, and garlic. Add the red onion and stir. Set aside.

Pat the fish dry and rub with the remaining 1 tablespoon (15 ml) olive oil. Season with Old Bay. Place on the prepared sheet pan. Bake for 12 to 15 minutes, until flaky.

Add the cherry tomatoes, cannellini beans, and parsley to the dressing mixture. Fold in the cheese. Refrigerate until the fish is cooked and you are ready to serve.

Divide the salad among four plates, add one-quarter of the baked fish to each, and serve.

NOTES

- **Tips:** If you're prepping ahead of time, keep the dressing mixture separate from the tomato, beans, and parsley mixture until you are ready to serve.

- **Easy Swaps:** To add heft (and omega-3s) to this meal, replace the white fish with salmon.

NUTRITIONAL ANALYSIS

SERVING SIZE: 6 ounces (170 g) fish, 2 cups (200 g) salad

PER SERVING: 462 calories; 19 g fat; 42 g protein; 26 g carbohydrates; 8 g fiber

SHEET-PAN COD DINNER

YIELD:
4 SERVINGS

PREP TIME:
5 MINUTES

COOK TIME:
30 MINUTES

Working fish into your eating pattern at least once per week can help to improve your metabolism and insulin sensitivity and can lower your risk of heart disease, so this sheet-pan meal deserves a place on your menu. Potatoes can get a bad rep, but they're high in fiber, potassium, and other essential nutrients; they absolutely can be part of a balanced meal.

1 pound (450 g) Yukon gold potatoes, cut into ½-inch (1.3 cm) pieces

1 medium-size yellow onion, chopped

2 tablespoons (30 ml) olive oil

1 teaspoon fresh thyme leaves

½ teaspoon salt, plus more as needed

¼ teaspoon black pepper, plus more as needed

12 ounces (340 g) fresh green beans

1½ pounds (680 g) cod

¾ cup (60 g) whole-grain breadcrumbs

1 tablespoon (2 g) chopped fresh parsley

2 teaspoons (2 g) Italian seasoning

2 tablespoons (30 g) unsalted butter, melted

1 teaspoon lemon zest

Preheat the oven to 425°F (220°C). Line an 18 by 13-inch (45 by 33 cm) sheet pan with parchment paper.

Combine the potatoes and onion in a mixing bowl and toss with 1 tablespoon (15 ml) of the olive oil, the thyme, and ¼ teaspoon of the salt, and black pepper. Transfer the mixture to the prepared sheet pan and evenly spread out. Roast for 10 minutes.

Meanwhile, in the same mixing bowl, combine the green beans, the remaining 1 tablespoon (15 ml) olive oil, and remaining ¼ teaspoon salt. After the potatoes have roasted for 10 minutes, slide the potatoes to one side of the pan and spread the green beans on the other side. Roast for 5 minutes more.

Cut the cod into four (6-ounce/170 g) portions. Pat each dry. Season lightly with salt and pepper.

Combine the breadcrumbs, parsley, Italian seasoning, melted butter, and lemon zest in a small bowl and mix well. Press one-quarter of the mixture firmly on top of each cod filet.

Slide the green beans and potatoes over on the pan to make room and add the cod. Roast for 14 to 15 minutes more, until the cod is cooked through and flaky. Serve immediately.

NUTRITIONAL ANALYSIS

SERVING SIZE: 6 ounces (170 g) cod, 3 ounces (85 g) green beans, ¾ cup (170 g) potatoes

PER SERVING: 427 calories; 14 g fat; 36 g protein; 38 g carbohydrates; 5 g fiber

NOTES

- **Tips:** If you don't have a half sheet pan, roast the vegetables on one quarter sheet pan and the cod on another. Large sheet pans come in handy, though, so I recommend investing in one.

- **Easy Swaps:** Halibut or pollock both make good replacements for cod.

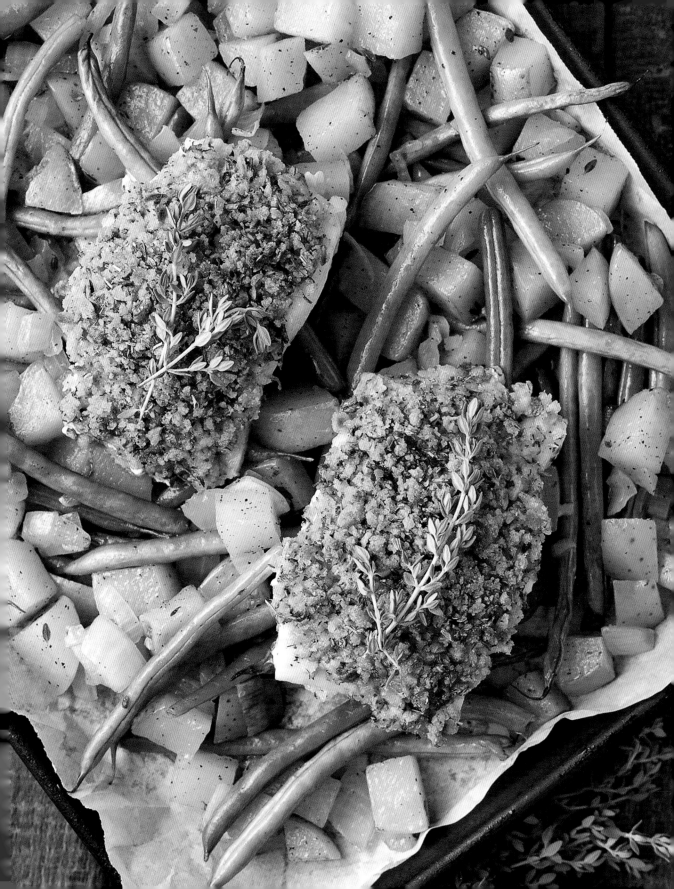

GREEK-STYLE SALMON BOWL

This grain bowl delivers heart-healthy fats, quality protein, and plenty of fiber, making it easy for you to pull together a healthy weeknight meal without sacrificing taste. It's fine to use frozen fruits and vegetables, like the green beans here. They're harvested and frozen at peak ripeness to lock in nutrients, making them a convenient, affordable, and nutrient-dense choice.

■ **YIELD:**
4 SERVINGS

■ **PREP TIME:**
10 MINUTES

■ **COOK TIME:**
25 MINUTES

1 cup (200 g) farro

1¼ pounds (570 g) salmon fillet

2 tablespoons (30 ml) olive or avocado oil, plus more as needed

¼ teaspoon salt, plus more as needed

¼ teaspoon black pepper, plus more as needed

4 cups (400 g) frozen cut green beans

3 tablespoons (45 ml) lemon juice

1 teaspoon minced garlic

½ teaspoon dried oregano

2 Roma tomatoes, chopped

½ cup (75 g) crumbled feta cheese

Preheat the oven to 400°F (200°F). Line an 18 by 13-inch (45 by 33 cm) sheet pan with parchment paper.

Bring 3 cups (720 ml) of water and 1 teaspoon of salt to a boil in a medium saucepan. Add the farro, partially cover, reduce the heat to medium-high and cook for 25 minutes until tender. Drain off any excess water.

Meanwhile, place the salmon on the prepared baking sheet, rub lightly with oil, and sprinkle with the salt and pepper. Bake for 15 to 18 minutes, until the salmon is opaque, then remove from the oven and let rest for 5 minutes.

Steam the green beans in a steamer basket over 1 inch (2.5 cm) of water on the stove for about 5 minutes, or microwave with 1 tablespoon (15 ml) of water for 3 minutes. If using frozen green beans in a steamer bag, microwave according to package directions.

Whisk together lemon juice, 2 tablespoons (30 ml) oil, garlic, oregano, and a pinch of salt in a small bowl.

To assemble, divide the farro among four plates. Arrange equal portions of the salmon, green beans, tomatoes, and feta cheese on top of the farro, drizzle with the dressing, and serve.

NUTRITIONAL ANALYSIS

SERVING SIZE: 5 ounces (140 g) salmon, one-quarter of the veggies and grains

PER SERVING: 514 calories; 20 g fat; 43 g protein; 8 g carbohydrates; 6 g fiber

NOTES

- **Tips:** Farro is an easy-to-prepare and versatile whole grain that can be used in just about any recipe in place of quinoa or rice.

- **Easy Swap:** Swapping roasted red peppers for the tomatoes brings a different but equally delicious flavor profile to this recipe.

LOADED COBB SALAD

There's nothing wrong with the original Cobb salad, which serves up protein-rich chicken, eggs, and bacon surrounded by avocado and blue cheese, all on a bed of greens. But I spruce up mine with cannellini beans, hemp seeds, and even more chicken (extra fiber and protein) for a filling meal that promotes insulin sensitivity.

■ YIELD:
4 SERVINGS

■ PREP TIME:
10 MINUTES

■ COOK TIME:
15 MINUTES

■ ASSEMBLY TIME:
5 MINUTES

4 cups (560 g) cubed raw chicken breast

1 tablespoon (15 ml) olive oil

Salt and black pepper

4 large eggs, hard-boiled and peeled

4 slices bacon

8 cups (240 g) coarsely chopped romaine lettuce

2 medium tomatoes, chopped

2 green onions, light and dark green parts only, sliced

1 cup (140 g) blue cheese crumbles

1 cup (165 g) canned cannellini beans, drained and rinsed

4 tablespoons (40 g) hemp seeds

1 large avocado, pitted, peeled, and sliced

8 tablespoons (120 g) yogurt-based ranch dressing

To prep the proteins (this can easily be done in advance), season the chicken cubes with salt and pepper and stir-fry in a large skillet with 1 tablespoon (15 ml) olive oil over medium-high heat until the chicken reaches an internal temperature of 165°F (75°C) and no pink remains. Finely chop the eggs. Cook the bacon in a skillet over medium heat until crispy, drain off the fat and pat dry, and let cool. Crumble the bacon into small bits.

To assemble the salads, split the lettuce among four bowls. Top each with equal portions of eggs, bacon, chicken, tomatoes, green onions, blue cheese, beans, hemp seeds, and avocado. Drizzle each with 2 tablespoons (30 ml) of dressing before serving.

NOTES

- **Tips:** Cook the proteins for this salad whenever you have time so you can whip it up on busy weeknights. You can also keep grilled frozen chicken breasts in the freezer to speed things up; just microwave according to package directions.

- **Easy Swap:** Cannellini beans can be swapped with black beans or chickpeas.

NUTRITIONAL ANALYSIS

SERVING SIZE: 1 salad

PER SERVING: 688 calories; 40 g fat; 59 g protein; 22 g carbohydrates; 9 g fiber

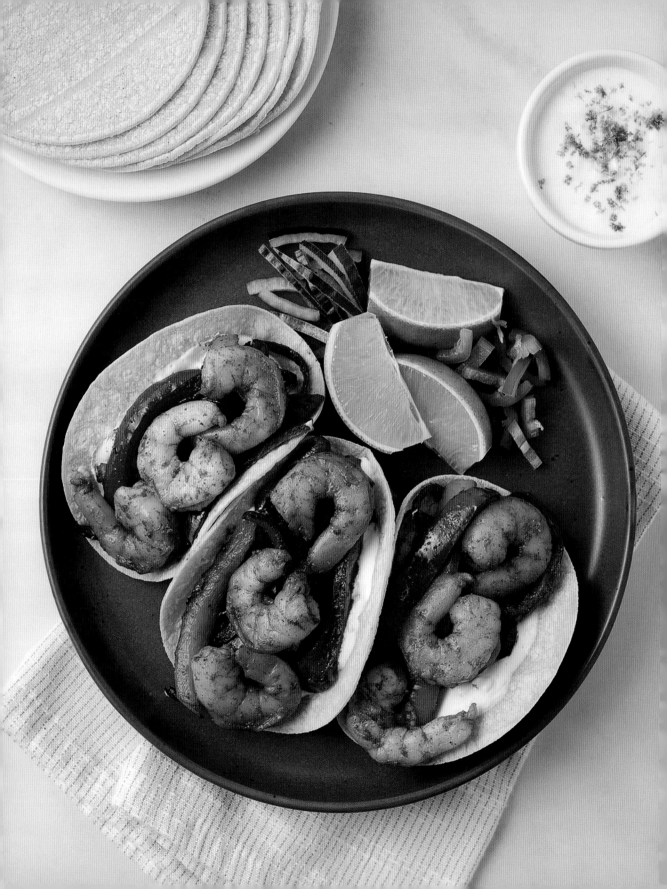

20-MINUTE SHEET-PAN TACOS

There's nothing simpler to prepare and easier to clean up than a sheet-pan dish. Try this one and you'll have a gluten-free dinner on the table in less than half an hour. An added plus: Shrimp are one of the leanest protein sources in the world.

■ YIELD:
4 SERVINGS

■ PREP TIME:
5 MINUTES

■ COOK TIME:
15 MINUTES

1¼ pounds (570 g) raw peeled and deveined large shrimp

1 red bell pepper, seeded and sliced

1 orange bell pepper, seeded and sliced

1 poblano pepper, seeded and sliced

1 red onion, sliced

3 tablespoons (45 ml) olive oil

1 tablespoon (8 g) chili powder

1 teaspoon ground cumin

½ teaspoon ground coriander

½ teaspoon salt

¾ cup (180 g) plain nonfat Greek yogurt

1 tablespoon (10 g) finely chopped jalapeño

¼ teaspoon lime zest

1 tablespoon (15 ml) fresh lime juice

1 teaspoon minced garlic

12 small (4½ inch/11.5 cm) corn tortillas

Preheat the oven to 400°F (200°C). Line a 9½ by 13-inch (24 by 33 cm) sheet pan with foil.

Toss together the shrimp, bell peppers, poblano pepper, onion, olive oil, chili powder, cumin, coriander, and ¼ teaspoon of the salt. Spread out on the prepared baking sheet.

Bake for 9 to 10 minutes until the shrimp are opaque. Remove the shrimp and wrap them in foil to keep warm. Turn the broiler to high and place the veggies back in the oven on the top rack to broil 3 to 4 minutes, or until they are slightly browned.

Meanwhile, stir together the yogurt, jalapeño, lime zest and juice, garlic, and the remaining ¼ teaspoon of salt in a small bowl to make a sauce. Warm the tortillas on a skillet for 1 minute each side. Wrap the tortillas in a clean kitchen towel and keep warm in the oven until serving.

To serve, spread the sauce on the tortillas and top with equal portions of veggies and shrimp.

NOTES

- **Tip:** Make this one-pan wonder even faster by prepping the sauce and veggies up to 2 days in advance.

- **Easy Swap:** Swap out the shrimp for an equal amount of white fish, chicken, or cubed and marinated tofu.

NUTRITIONAL ANALYSIS

SERVING SIZE: 3 tacos

PER SERVING: 414 calories; 14 g fat; 35 g protein; 35 g carbohydrates; 4 g fiber

BALANCED BURRITO BOWLS

This kid-friendly meal is a healthier version of the popular takeout treat. It's the perfect crowd-pleaser, too, since you can easily double or triple the batch if you're cooking for a big group. Plus, this combination of ingredients helps to stabilize blood sugar and reduce insulin spikes.

■ **YIELD:**
4 SERVINGS

■ **PREP TIME:**
10 MINUTES

■ **COOK TIME:**
15 MINUTES

■ **ASSEMBLY TIME:**
5 MINUTES

FOR THE CILANTRO-LIME RICE

2 cups (480 ml) water

¼ teaspoon salt

1 cup (185 g) uncooked basmati or jasmine rice, rinsed

1 tablespoon (15 ml) lime juice

¼ cup (10 g) chopped fresh cilantro

FOR THE SEASONING

2 teaspoons (5 g) onion powder

1 tablespoon plus 1 teaspoon (10 g) paprika

1 tablespoon (8 g) chili powder

1 teaspoon ground cumin

1 teaspoon garlic powder

½ teaspoon salt

¼ teaspoon black pepper

¼ teaspoon white pepper

FOR THE BOWLS

1 (15-ounce/400 g) can black beans, drained and rinsed

¼ cup (60 ml) water

2 large boneless, skinless chicken breasts

1 tablespoon (15 ml) olive oil

1½ cups (225 g) cherry tomatoes, halved

1½ cups (200 g) frozen corn, thawed

4 ounces (115 g) shredded cheddar cheese

2 cups (120 g) romaine lettuce, cut into thin ribbons

To make the rice, bring the water and salt to a boil in a saucepan. Add the rice, cover, and cook for about 15 minutes, until tender. Add the lime juice and cilantro, stir, and set aside.

To make the seasoning. Combine the onion powder, paprika, chili powder, cumin, garlic powder, salt, black pepper, and white pepper in a small bowl.

To make the bowls, in a small saucepan over medium heat, combine the black beans with 1 tablespoon (15 ml) of the seasoning and the water. Mix, bring to a boil, then remove from heat and cover to keep warm.

Cut the chicken breasts in half horizontally to make four thinner cutlets. Use the remaining seasoning to coat the chicken on both sides. Heat the olive oil in a large skillet over medium-high heat, add the chicken, and cook for about 4 minutes per side, until cooked through with no pink remaining, or until they reach an internal temperature of 165°F (75°C).

To make the guacamole, pit the avocados, scoop out the flesh with a spoon, mash with a fork in a bowl. Add the lime juice, cilantro, onion, and garlic salt. Mix to combine.

Assemble the bowls by dividing the rice among four bowls. Top each with equal portions of chicken, tomatoes, corn, cheddar cheese, lettuce, beans, and 2 tablespoons (60 g) of guacamole (you will have guacamole left over).

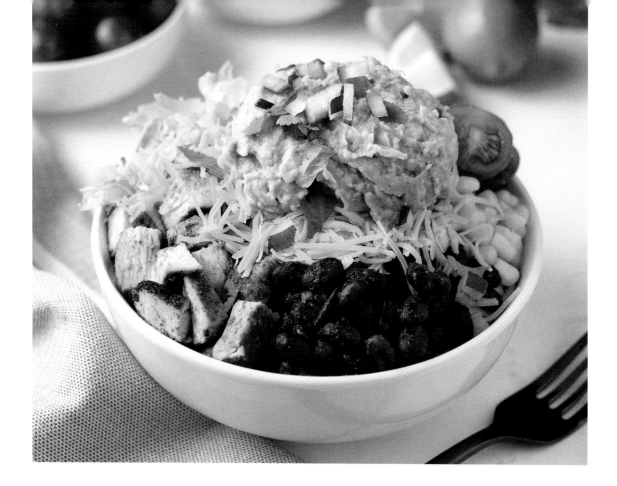

FOR THE GUACAMOLE

3 avocados

2 tablespoons (30 ml) lime juice

2 tablespoons (10 g) chopped
fresh cilantro

2 tablespoons (15 g) chopped
red onion

Garlic salt

NOTES

- **Tips:** This recipe is perfect for advance meal prep. I recommend keeping the beans, corn, and chicken in separate bowls for reheating, adding them to the bowl with the rest of the ingredients when serving.

- **Easy Swaps:** Use this recipe as a template and swap the chicken for steak (or your preferred protein), and switch out the veggies and/or cheese for your favorites.

NUTRITIONAL ANALYSIS

SERVING SIZE: 1 bowl

PER SERVING: 650 calories;
18 g fat; 49 g protein;
76 g carbohydrates; 12 g fiber

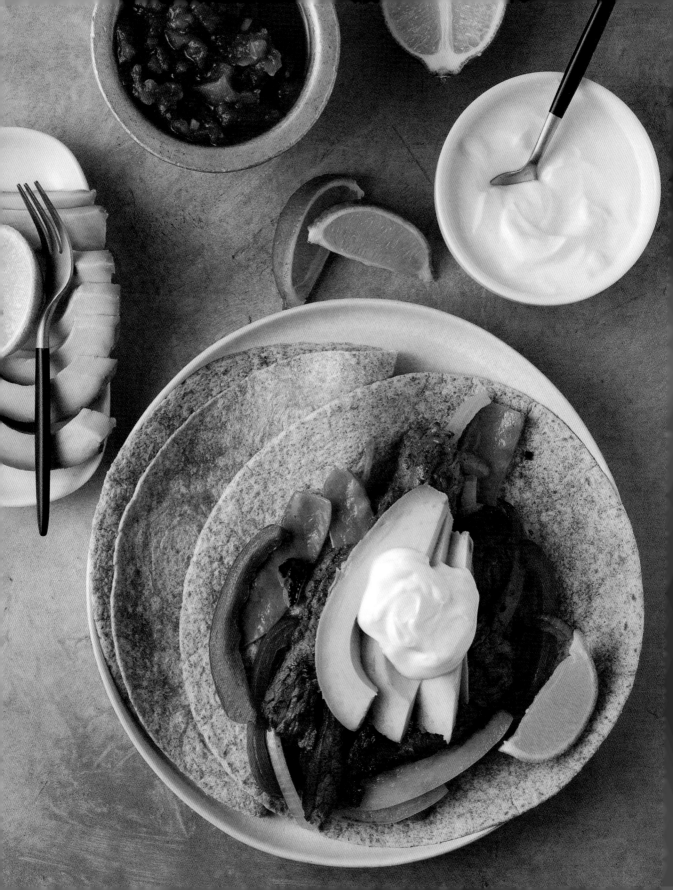

VEGGIE-BOOSTED STEAK FAJITAS

My Tex-Mex favorite packs extra veggies for fiber, stir-fried in avocado oil for a crisp-tender texture. Yes, you can have red meat! Less than 25 grams of saturated fat daily supports insulin sensitivity—and this dish has just 6 grams per serving!

YIELD:
4 SERVINGS

PREP TIME:
20 MINUTES

COOK TIME:
15 MINUTES

1½ pounds (680 g) sirloin steak or flank steak

1 tablespoon (7 g) chili powder

2 teaspoons (4 g) ground cumin

1 teaspoon paprika

Salt and black pepper

3 cloves garlic, minced

1 red bell pepper

1 yellow bell pepper

1 medium-size yellow onion

¼ cup (60 ml) avocado oil

1½ cups (150 g) snow peas

8 (6-inch/15 cm) whole-wheat tortillas

1 avocado, peeled, pitted, and sliced (optional)

2 tablespoons (30 g) plain nonfat Greek yogurt (optional)

Pat the steak dry and let rest on a plate for about 20 minutes to bring to room temperature.

Meanwhile, mix the chili powder, cumin, paprika, and a pinch each of salt and pepper in a small bowl. Add the minced garlic and combine. Rub onto the steak on both sides and let the meat rest while you thinly slice the red pepper, yellow pepper, and onion.

Heat 2 tablespoons (30 ml) of avocado oil in a high-sided skillet or wok over medium-high heat. Add all the vegetables and stir until coated, then season to taste with salt and pepper. Stir-fry, uncovered, for about 12 minutes, or until the veggies are crisp-tender.

Meanwhile, heat 2 tablespoons (30 ml) of avocado oil in a large cast-iron skillet over medium-high heat (or preheat a grill to medium-high heat). Cook the steak for 4 to 5 minutes per side, to your desired doneness.

Gently wipe the grease from the steak skillet with a paper towel, leaving about 1 tablespoon (15 ml) of grease in the pan and return the heat to medium-high. Warm the tortillas in the skillet for about 1 minute per side.

Thinly slice the steak. Divide the steak and veggies among the warm tortillas and top each with sliced avocado and Greek yogurt.

NOTES

- **Tips:** Control the amount of saturated fat in recipes that call for red meat by choosing a lean cut.

- **Easy Swaps:** Like your fajitas spicy? Add your favorite hot sauce or a chimichurri sauce. Using plain Greek yogurt in place of sour cream adds the same great tang plus a boost of protein, but if you're not a fan, low-fat sour cream works just fine.

NUTRITIONAL ANALYSIS

SERVING SIZE: 2 fajitas

PER SERVING: 378 calories; 24 g fat; 45 g protein; 46 g carbohydrates; 7 g fiber

LETTUCE WRAPS WITH SAVORY GINGER RICE

■ **YIELD:**
6 SERVINGS

■ **PREP TIME:**
10 MINUTES

■ **COOK TIME:**
15 MINUTES

My spin on the lettuce wraps beloved by fans of a certain popular Chinese restaurant is lower in sugar and sodium, but packs just as much flavor. Better yet? Way more fiber. Serve this dish family-style so everyone can assemble their own lettuce wraps.

FOR THE SAVORY GINGER RICE

- 1 cup (185 g) jasmine or basmati rice
- 1⅛ cups (265 ml) water
- 2 teaspoons (10 ml) rice vinegar
- 1 teaspoon ground ginger
- ⅛ teaspoon salt
- 1 green onion, both green and white parts, thinly sliced

To make the ginger rice, rinse the rice in a mesh strainer until it becomes slightly translucent. Combine the rice, water, rice vinegar, ginger, salt, and green onions in a pot. Cook according to package directions. Alternatively, add all the ingredients to a rice cooker and cook according to its directions.

NOTES

- **Tip:** If you don't have a mesh strainer for rinsing the rice, add the rice directly to the pot, add water to cover, and swish the rice around. Once the water is cloudy, pour it off. Repeat this two to three times, or until the water runs mostly clear.

- **Easy Swaps:** To kick up the spice level, swap the red bell pepper with a red jalapeño or another spicy pepper. Gochujang, a Korean red chili paste, can be found in the Asian section of most grocery stores, but if you can't find it, substitute 1 teaspoon sriracha sauce.

NUTRITIONAL ANALYSIS

SERVING SIZE: ⅔ cup (133 g) rice, ¼ pound (115 g) pork mixture

PER SERVING: 539 calories; 29 g fat; 35 g protein; 32 g carbohydrates; 3 g fiber

FOR THE LETTUCE WRAPS

- 1 tablespoon (15 ml) toasted sesame oil
- ½ medium-size red bell pepper, chopped
- ½ cup (60 g) shredded carrot
- ½ cup (50 g) diced celery
- 2 green onions, chopped, green and white parts separated
- 1½ pounds (680 g) ground pork
- 3 tablespoons (45 ml) low-sodium soy sauce
- 1 tablespoon (16 g) natural sugar-free peanut butter
- 1 tablespoon (21 g) honey
- 1 tablespoon (15 ml) rice vinegar
- 1 tablespoon (15 g) gochujang (chili paste)
- 1 teaspoon minced garlic
- 1 teaspoon sesame seeds
- ½ teaspoon ground ginger
- 2 heads butter lettuce
- ¼ cup (30 g) cashews, or other nuts of your choice
- 1 medium-size avocado, pitted, peeled, and sliced

To make the wraps, heat the sesame oil in a large skillet over medium heat. Add the red pepper, carrot, celery, and green onion whites and stir-fry for 4 minutes. Add the ground pork and cook for about 8 minutes until browned, stirring occasionally and breaking the meat into smaller pieces.

Meanwhile, whisk together the soy sauce, peanut butter, honey, rice vinegar, gochujang, garlic, sesame seeds, and ginger in a small bowl to make a sauce.

Reduce the heat under the pork mixture to medium. Add the onion greens and sauce to the pan. Cook for 2 minutes, or until the sauce reduces by about half.

Serve the butter lettuce, meat mixture, nuts, and avocado family style with the rice on the side. To make a wrap, put a thin slice of avocado and a few cashews on a leaf of lettuce. Spoon about 2 tablespoons (30 g) of the meat mixture onto the lettuce leaf. Fold and eat. Repeat and enjoy.

SMOKY ROMESCO WHITE BEANS WITH ROASTED BROCCOLINI

■ **YIELD:**
6 SERVINGS

■ **PREP TIME:**
15 MINUTES

■ **COOK TIME:**
20 MINUTES

This nutrient-packed vegetarian main pairs smoky romesco sauce with creamy white beans and crispy broccolini for a perfect balance of flavors and textures. The homemade romesco sauce is the star here, bringing a rich intensity to the beans.

FOR THE ROASTED BROCCOLINI

1½ pounds (675 g) broccolini
1½ tablespoons (22 ml) olive oil
Pinch of salt
Pinch of black pepper

Preheat the oven to 425°F (220°C). Line a 9½ by 13-inch (24 by 33 cm) sheet pan with parchment paper.

To make the broccolini, arrange it on the prepared baking sheet in a single layer. Drizzle with the olive oil and sprinkle with salt and pepper. Roast for 20 minutes, until crispy and lightly browned.

NOTES

- **Tips:** If you don't have a nonstick skillet, add the sauce to the pan before adding the beans: This will prevent them from sticking to the pan. Tahini can vary significantly in flavor by brand. I like the Mighty Sesame brand because it has a mellow flavor and comes in a squeezable bottle.

- **Easy Swaps:** You can swap out the maple syrup for the sugar-free maple-flavored variety, but it lends a nice sweetness to the romesco, and it adds less than 1 gram of sugar per serving, so consider leaving it in. If you can't find broccolini, fresh broccoli florets work just as well.

NUTRITIONAL ANALYSIS

SERVING SIZE: ¾ cup (360 g) romesco beans, 1 pita, ½ cup (40 g) broccolini

PER SERVING: 580 calories; 14 g fat; 26 g protein; 82 g carbohydrates, 15 g fiber

FOR THE ROMESCO WHITE BEANS

1 red bell pepper

1 (14.5-ounce/415 g) can fire-roasted tomatoes

½ cup (55 g) walnut pieces, divided

1 tablespoon plus 1 teaspoon (16 g) minced garlic

2 tablespoons (30 g) tahini

1 tablespoon (15 ml) apple cider vinegar

2 teaspoons (2 g) dried parsley

2 teaspoons (2 g) smoked paprika

¼ teaspoon cayenne pepper (optional)

1 teaspoon maple syrup

½ teaspoon salt

1 to 2 tablespoons (15 to 30 ml) water (optional)

2 (15-ounce/400 g) cans cannellini beans, drained and rinsed

FOR SERVING

6 whole-grain pita breads or whole-grain croutons

To make the Romesco white beans, place the red bell pepper directly over a gas flame using metal tongs, turning until charred on all sides, about 6 minutes. Alternatively, place it on a small skillet over high heat until charred on all sides. Cut in half, remove the stem and seeds, and coarsely chop.

In a blender or food processor, combine the roasted tomatoes, red pepper, walnuts, garlic, tahini, apple cider vinegar, parsley, smoked paprika, cayenne, if using, maple syrup, and salt. Blend for about 1 minute, until creamy and slightly runny, scraping the sides halfway through. Add water 1 teaspoon at a time to reach your desired consistency, if necessary.

Put a high-sided nonstick skillet and over medium heat and add the beans. Warm for 3 minutes, then add the romesco sauce. Continue warming for about 5 minutes more, until the sauce is heated through.

Serve the broccolini with whole-grain pita bread for dipping and scooping the romesco sauce. Garnish each serving with 1 tablespoon (7 g) of walnut pieces.

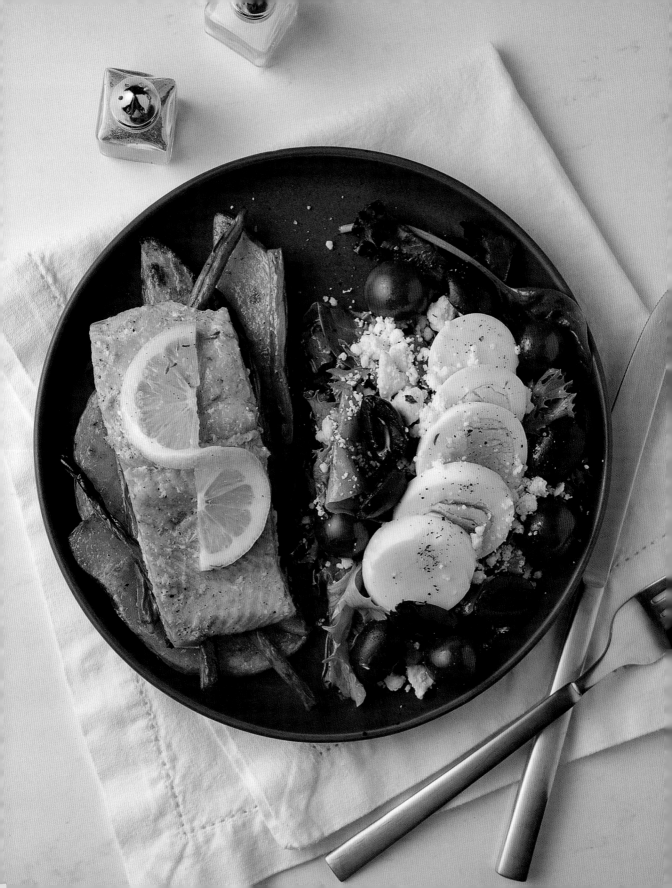

NIÇOISE SALAD WITH SALMON

Here's my take on a Niçoise salad. I've amped up the fiber and reduced the saturated fat content to promote insulin sensitivity. Salmon is an excellent source of those omega-3 fatty acids that are so important for metabolic health and brain function.

▓ **YIELD:**
4 SERVINGS

▓ **PREP TIME:**
5 MINUTES

▓ **COOK TIME:**
25 MINUTES

▓ **ASSEMBLY TIME:**
5 MINUTES

FOR THE SALAD

- 2 cups (200 g) fresh green beans, trimmed
- 2 cups (300 g) unpeeled, wedged Yukon gold potatoes
- 2 tablespoons plus 2 teaspoons (40 ml) olive oil, divided
- Salt and black pepper
- 1½ pounds (680 g) salmon fillet
- 12 cups (300 g) mixed salad greens
- 4 large eggs, hard-boiled, peeled, and sliced
- 2 cups (300 g) cherry tomatoes
- ½ cup (75 g) crumbled feta cheese
- ½ cup (75 g) kalamata olives (optional)

FOR THE LEMON VINAIGRETTE

- ½ cup (120 ml) olive oil
- 2 tablespoons (30 ml) lemon juice
- ½ teaspoon minced garlic
- ¼ teaspoon dried thyme
- Pinch of salt
- Pinch of black pepper

NUTRITIONAL ANALYSIS

SERVING SIZE: 6 ounces (170 g) salmon, 4 cups (400 g) veggies

PER SERVING: 375 calories; 42 g fat; 33 g protein; 15 g carbohydrates; 6 g fiber

Preheat the oven to 425°F (220°C). Line two 9½ by 13-inch (24 by 33 cm) sheet pans with parchment paper.

To make the salad, toss the green beans and potato wedges with 2 tablespoons (30 ml) olive oil, salt, and pepper. Spread out on one of the prepared sheet pans and roast for 25 minutes.

Meanwhile, prepare the salmon: Pat dry, rub lightly with the remaining olive oil, and season with salt and pepper. Place on the second prepared sheet pan and roast for 15 minutes, or until opaque and flaky.

To make the vinaigrette, combine the olive oil, lemon juice, garlic, thyme, salt, and pepper in a small jar and shake to combine, or whisk in a bowl.

To assemble the salads, divide the salad greens among four plates, pushing them to one side. Top each with a sliced hard-boiled egg, one-quarter of the cherry tomatoes, feta cheese, and kalamata olives, if using. Add one-quarter of the potatoes, one-quarter of the green beans, and 6 ounces (170 g) salmon to each plate. Drizzle with the vinaigrette and serve immediately.

NOTES

- **Tip:** If you're making this ahead and saving some for leftovers, be sure to use within 3 days and store the dressing separately.

- **Easy Swaps:** If you're not a fan of olives, simply omit them or substitute roasted red peppers or pickled beets. Instead of wedged Yukon gold potatoes, you can use 2 cups (350 g) baby potatoes, halved.

CHICKEN AND CHICKPEA SALAD

YIELD:
4 SERVINGS

PREP TIME:
10 MINUTES

COOK TIME:
10 MINUTES

Every portion of this Mediterranean-style salad offers three full servings of vegetables and a very satisfying combination of textures, not to mention multiple protein sources. Got leftovers? Extra portions make great workday lunches (see note).

1 cup (100 g) uncooked whole-wheat rotini pasta

¼ cup (60 ml) avocado oil

2 tablespoons (30 ml) red wine vinegar

¼ teaspoon celery salt

8 cups (240 g) spring greens

1 (15-ounce/400 g) can chickpeas, drained and rinsed

1 (10-ounce/280 g) can chicken breast, drained

1 cup (150 g) cherry tomatoes, halved

1 cup (150 g) crumbled feta cheese

1 cup (140 g) kalamata olives (optional)

Cook the pasta according to package directions. Drain well.

Make the dressing by whisking together the avocado oil, vinegar, and celery salt.

Add one-quarter of the greens to each of four salad bowls. Top each with equal portions of chickpeas, chicken, cooked pasta, cherry tomatoes, feta, olives, and about 1½ tablespoons (20 ml) dressing.

NUTRITIONAL ANALYSIS

SERVING SIZE: 2 cups (100 g) greens, about ⅓ cup (55 g) chickpeas, ½ cup (110 g) pasta, one-quarter of the tomatoes, feta, olives, and dressing

PER SERVING: 560 calories; 29 g fat; 34 g protein; 40 g carbohydrates; 11 g fiber

NOTES

- **Tips:** If you're prepping this salad to enjoy later, layer each serving of this salad in a mason jar in this order: dressing, chickpeas, tomatoes, olives, pasta, feta, greens. This way it'll stay fresh in the refrigerator for up to 5 days.

- **Easy Swaps:** For a vegetarian option, ditch the chicken and use a total of 2½ cups (350 g) of chickpeas for extra protein. Or, use a higher-protein pasta: Many popular brands now offer versions made with pulses like lentils, peas, and chickpeas.

GOAT CHEESE AND RED PEPPER
TWICE-BAKED POTATOES WITH SPINACH

YIELD:
4 SERVINGS

PREP TIME:
20 MINUTES

COOK TIME:
75 MINUTES

Twice-baked potatoes are fun and blood sugar-friendly! Cooling and reheating them creates resistant starch, which digests more slowly, reducing glycemic impact. So go ahead and dig in!

FOR THE POTATOES

2 large russet potatoes

1 tablespoon (15 ml) olive oil

1 medium-size yellow onion, halved and very thinly sliced

½ cup (70 g) roasted red peppers in oil, drained and chopped

⅓ cup (45 g) soft goat cheese

¼ cup (60 ml) 2% low-fat milk

1 cup (140 g) shredded rotisserie chicken

¼ teaspoon salt

¼ teaspoon black pepper

FOR THE SPINACH

1 tablespoon (15 ml) olive oil

1 tablespoon (3 g) minced garlic

¼ teaspoon dried red pepper flakes

16 ounces (450 g) fresh baby spinach

1 tablespoon (15 ml) lemon juice

Salt

Preheat the oven to 400°F (200°C).

Scrub the potatoes, wrap each in aluminum foil, and bake for 60 minutes. Let cool completely and store in an airtight container in the refrigerator. This process can be done up to 3 days in advance.

Preheat the oven to 400°F (200°C). Line a 9½ by 13-inch (24 by 33 cm) sheet pan with parchment paper.

Heat the oil in a large skillet over medium heat. Add the onion and saute for 8 to 10 minutes, until caramelized. Add the red peppers and cook for 2 minutes. Remove from the heat.

Cut the potatoes in half lengthwise and scoop the flesh into a large mixing bowl, leaving a ¼-inch (6 mm) shell. Add the goat cheese, milk, chicken, salt, pepper, and cooked onion and red pepper mix to the bowl. Use a hand mixer to mix until just combined. Use a large spoon to scoop the filling back into the potato shells and place on the sheet pan.

Bake for 15 minutes. If you like, turn the broiler to high and broil for the last 2 minutes of baking to brown the tops of the potatoes.

When 6 to 8 minutes remain, sauté the spinach in the skillet used for the onions over medium heat. Add the olive oil. When hot, add the garlic and red pepper flakes. Add the spinach, cover, and cook for about 5 minutes, or until wilted, stirring halfway through. Remove from the heat and add lemon juice and salt, stirring just until mixed in.

Serve the spinach immediately alongside a twice-baked potato half.

NUTRITIONAL ANALYSIS

SERVING SIZE: ½ potato with filling, ¼ cup (60 g) sauteed spinach

PER SERVING: 328 calories; 11 g fat; 20 g protein; 36 g carbohydrates; 6 g fiber

MEDITERRANEAN CUCUMBER AND TOMATO GRAIN BOWLS

YIELD:
4 SERVINGS

PREP TIME:
15 MINUTES

ASSEMBLY TIME:
5 MINUTES

Make these light and refreshing grain bowls on warm summer evenings when you don't feel like turning on the oven. They're packed with plant-based protein thanks to chickpeas and quinoa and can be turned into a quick meal by adding just about any combination of veggies. I love the Greek-style flavors here—olives, hummus, and tzatziki—and the fact that it only takes twenty minutes to get it to the table.

FOR THE VEGETABLE MIXTURE

1 cucumber, chopped

2 cups (300 g) cherry tomatoes, halved

2 green onions, light and dark green parts only, sliced

½ cup (15 g) chopped fresh parsley

1 tablespoon plus 1 teaspoon (20 ml) olive oil

1 tablespoon (15 ml) red wine vinegar

Pinch of salt

FOR THE BOWLS

¾ cup (120 g) uncooked quinoa

1 (15-ounce/400 g) can chickpeas, drained and rinsed

1 cup (150 g) kalamata olives

1 cup (240 g) hummus

½ cup (120 g) tzatziki sauce

Black pepper

To prepare the vegetable mixture, toss the cucumber, tomatoes, green onions, and parsley in a large mixing bowl with the oil, vinegar, and pinch of salt. Set aside.

To prepare the bowls, cook the quinoa according to package directions.

To assemble the bowls, divide the cooked quinoa, vegetable mixture, chickpeas, and olives among four bowls. Top each with ¼ cup (60 g) hummus and 2 tablespoons (30 g) tzatziki, garnish with black pepper, and serve.

NOTES

- **Tip:** These grain bowls are just as good for lunch as they are for dinner, so prep them ahead and get lunch for the week taken care of. They'll stay fresh in the fridge for up to 5 days.

- **Easy Swaps:** You can swap the chickpeas with chicken, or simply add a serving of chicken, if you need extra protein.

NUTRITIONAL ANALYSIS

SERVING SIZE: 1 bowl

PER SERVING: 546 calories; 22 g fat; 21 g protein; 66 g carbohydrates; 17 g fiber

KALE- AND MUSHROOM-STUFFED PASTA SHELLS

■ YIELD:
4 SERVINGS

■ PREP TIME:
10 MINUTES

■ COOK TIME:
25 MINUTES

Pasta shells are blank canvases; you can stuff them with an abundance of nutritious fillings. In this vegetarian recipe, I manage to cram a full serving of vegetables and protein into each portion without going overboard on carbohydrates.

20 jumbo pasta shells (from a 12-ounce/340 g box)

2 cups (480 g) no-sugar-added red pasta sauce

2 cups (160 g) diced white mushrooms

1½ cups (45 g) finely chopped lacinato kale

2 cups (480 g) low-fat cottage cheese

½ cup (50 g) grated Parmesan cheese

1 cup (120 g) shredded low-fat mozzarella

¼ teaspoon salt

Cook the pasta according to the package directions, or until slightly softer than al dente. Drain in a colander, then dip in ice-cold water to cool quickly. Drain again and set aside.

Preheat the oven to 400°F (200°F). Coat a 9 by 13-inch (23 by 33 cm) baking dish with cooking spray. Spread the pasta sauce evenly across the bottom.

Mix the mushrooms, kale, cottage cheese, Parmesan, ½ cup (60 g) of the shredded mozzarella, and salt in a large bowl, stirring until combined.

Use a spoon to stuff each of the pasta shells with about 3 tablespoons (45 g) of the cheese and vegetable mixture. They should be overstuffed.

Arrange the stuffed shells in a single layer in the baking dish. Top with the remaining ½ cup (60 g) of mozzarella. Bake for 10 minutes. Then turn the broiler on high and broil on the top rack for 2 to 3 minutes more, until mozzarella on top is slightly browned.

Let cool 5 minutes before serving. Store leftovers in the refrigerator for up to 5 days.

NOTES

- **Tip:** Stuffed shells are a fun way to enjoy a high-volume pasta meal without overloading on carbs.

- **Easy Swaps:** Curly kale or spinach also work well in this recipe. If you don't like mushrooms, try using chopped broccoli or cauliflower. It can be tough to find whole-grain jumbo pasta shells, but if you do find them, by all means use them.

NUTRITIONAL ANALYSIS

SERVING SIZE: 5 stuffed shells

PER SERVING: 455 calories; 13 g fat; 35 g protein; 53 g carbohydrates; 4 g fiber

SWEET AND SAVORY HARVEST SHEET-PAN DINNER

■ **YIELD:**
6 SERVINGS

■ **PREP TIME:**
15 MINUTES

■ **COOK TIME:**
25 MINUTES

I've included several sheet-pan dinners in this book because they're such a great way to mix flavors and textures into a no-fuss yet balanced meal, and this one is no exception. Maple-flavored syrup and cinnamon infuse this recipe with autumn flavor, but you don't have to wait 'til September to enjoy it. Make it year-round.

---

4 tablespoons (60 ml) olive oil

2 tablespoons (30 ml) sugar-free maple-flavored syrup

3 tablespoons (45 ml) apple cider vinegar

2 tablespoons (30 g) Dijon mustard

2 teaspoons (4 g) ground cumin

1 teaspoon chili powder

1 teaspoon paprika

½ teaspoon salt

½ teaspoon cayenne pepper

½ teaspoon ground cinnamon

2 large shallots, thinly sliced

1 pound (450 g) peeled and cubed butternut squash

24 ounces (680 g) brussels sprouts

1 large Honeycrisp apple, cored and cubed (do not peel)

2 large boneless, skinless chicken breasts, cubed

¼ teaspoon salt

¼ teaspoon black pepper

Preheat the oven to 425°F (220°C). Line a 18 by 13-inch (45 by 33 cm) sheet pan with parchment paper.

In a large jar, combine 3 tablespoons (45 ml) of the olive oil with the maple-flavored syrup, apple cider vinegar, Dijon mustard, cumin, chili powder, paprika, salt, cayenne, and cinnamon and shake well. Add the shallot to the jar and shake again. Set aside.

Combine the butternut squash, brussels sprouts, and cubed apple in a large bowl. Add the shallot dressing and toss to coat evenly. Spread the vegetables evenly on the baking sheet.

Place the chicken pieces in a separate bowl and toss with the remaining 1 tablespoon (15 ml) olive oil, salt, and pepper. Distribute the chicken pieces evenly among the vegetables. Roast for 20 to 25 minutes, stirring halfway through, or until the chicken is cooked through and the vegetables are crisp-tender. Serve hot.

NOTES

- **Tips:** This is a great recipe for meal prep, because it makes six full servings. If you are cooking for one or two, cutting the recipe in half is a good option. You can learn more about that in chapter 2.

- **Easy Swaps:** You can swap out brussels sprouts with broccoli and butternut squash with sweet potatoes.

NUTRITIONAL ANALYSIS

SERVING SIZE: 2 cups (410 g)

PER SERVING: 338 calories; 18 g fat; 18 g protein; 27 g carbohydrates; 6 g fiber

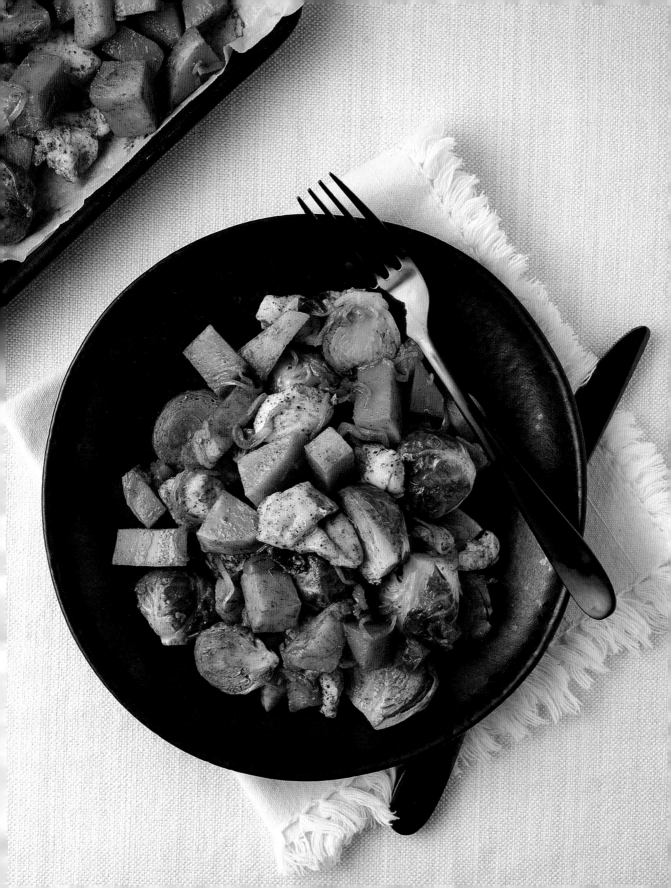

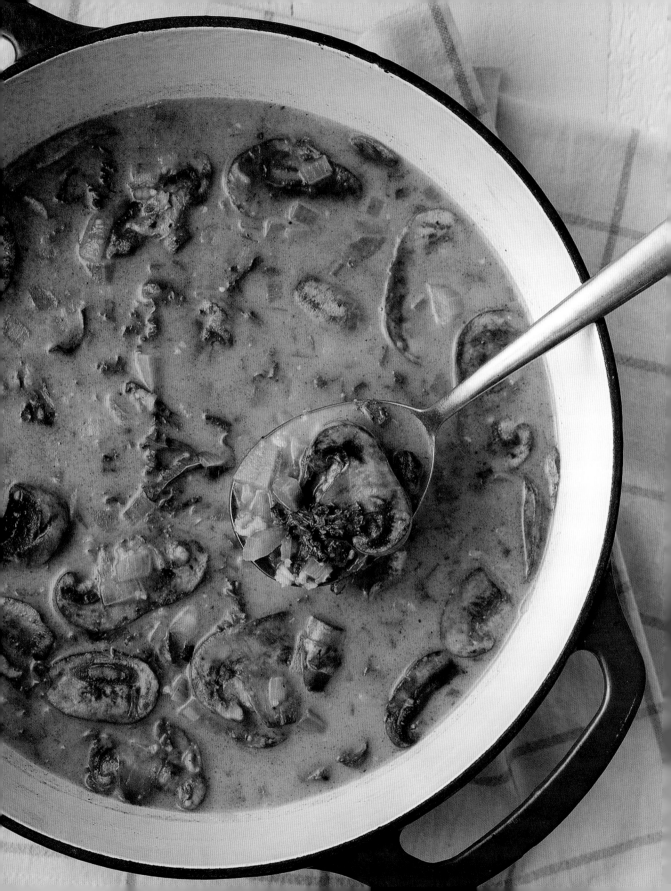

MEGAN'S CHICKEN, TAHINI, AND WILD RICE SOUP

YIELD:
6 SERVINGS

PREP TIME:
15 MINUTES

COOK TIME:
45 MINUTES

This isn't your average chicken soup. It's my all-time favorite, and my clients love how filling and comforting it is. It uses only whole ingredients and boasts a wide range of nutrients and good fats, thanks to sweet potatoes, carrots, celery, kale, and tahini. While the cooking time is on the long side, the active cooking time is low, so it's great for weeknights.

2 tablespoons (30 ml) olive oil

1 small white onion, diced

3 cloves garlic, minced

6 cups (1.4 L) low-sodium chicken broth

½ cup (100 g) uncooked wild rice

8 ounces (225 g) mushrooms, sliced

2 medium carrots, diced

2 stalks celery, diced

1 large sweet potato, peeled and diced

1 bay leaf

1½ tablespoons (9 g) Old Bay seasoning

1½ cups (180 g) shredded cooked chicken

1 cup (240 ml) 2% low-fat milk

¼ cup (60 g) tahini

2 cups (60 g) coarsely chopped kale

Salt and black pepper

Heat 1 tablespoon (15 ml) of the oil in a large soup pot over medium-high heat. Add the onion and saute for 4 minutes. Add garlic and saute for 1 minute more.

Add the chicken broth, wild rice, mushrooms, carrots, celery, sweet potato, bay leaf, and Old Bay seasoning. Stir to combine. Bring the soup to a simmer, then reduce the heat to medium-low and continue to simmer for 30 minutes, stirring occasionally,

Add the chicken to the soup. Whisk together the milk and tahini in a small bowl. Slowly add this to the soup and stir until combined. Then add the kale, stir, and add salt and pepper to taste. Cook for about 5 minutes more, until the rice and veggies are tender and the soup has cooked for 40 minutes. Serve hot.

NOTES

- **Tips:** The tahini and milk will separate quickly, so give the mixture an extra whisk right before adding it to the soup.

- **Easy Swaps:** Swap the sweet potatoes for butternut squash when it's in season.

NUTRITIONAL ANALYSIS

SERVING SIZE: 2 cups (485 g)

PER SERVING: 268 calories; 11 g fat; 17 g protein; 27 g carbohydrates; 5 g fiber

CREAMY TOMATO PASTA WITH TURKEY AND VEGGIES

This veggie- and protein-packed dinner is healthy comfort food at its very best. Whole-grain pasta contains fiber to help stabilize blood glucose, so it's a good choice as part of a high-protein meal like this one.

YIELD:
5 SERVINGS

PREP TIME:
5 MINUTES

COOK TIME:
20 MINUTES

- 8 ounces (225 g) uncooked whole-wheat rotini pasta
- 1 medium yellow onion, chopped
- 1½ pounds (680 g) ground turkey
- 1 tablespoon (15 ml) olive oil
- 8 ounces (225 g) mushrooms, sliced
- 1 medium-size zucchini, trimmed, quartered lengthwise, and chopped into ¼-inch (6 mm) thick pieces
- 2 cups (480 ml) no-sugar-added red pasta sauce
- 1 cup (240 ml) 2% low-fat milk
- 5 ounces (140 g) fresh baby spinach
- Salt (optional)
- Italian seasoning (optional)
- Garlic salt
- ½ cup (50 g) grated Parmesan cheese

Cook the pasta according to package directions. Drain well.

Place a large skillet over medium-high heat, add the onion and ground turkey, and cook until browned, about 7 minutes. Drain off any fat.

Meanwhile, add the oil to a separate large skillet over medium heat. Add the mushrooms and zucchini and saute until tender, about 6 minutes.

Add the pasta sauce and milk to the veggies and heat through, about 2 minutes. Add the spinach and cover the pan to allow it to wilt for 2 minutes. Stir well and taste for seasoning, adding the salt, Italian seasoning, and garlic salt as needed (see note below).

Add the turkey and cooked pasta to the sauce and veggies and stir until mixed well. Serve topped with a generous sprinkle of Parmesan cheese.

NOTES

- **Tips:** The flavor of this dish depends on the red sauce you choose, so pick your favorite. If you choose a basic red sauce and the flavor isn't quite what you want it to be, try adding 1 teaspoon of Italian seasoning and 1 teaspoon of garlic salt. Also, you can save time by buying pre-sliced mushrooms.

- **Easy Swaps:** Use kale, arugula, or even lettuce in place of the spinach and replace the mushrooms or zucchini with any veggies you prefer.

NUTRITIONAL ANALYSIS

SERVING SIZE: 2½ cups (475 g)

PER SERVING: 402 calories;
10 g fat; 49 g protein;
36 g carbohydrates; 9 g fiber

WHIPPED TAHINI TOFU WITH FARRO AND BALSAMIC VEGGIES

■ YIELD:
4 SERVINGS

■ PREP TIME:
10 MINUTES

■ COOK TIME:
20 MINUTES

■ ASSEMBLY TIME:
5 MINUTES

If you're new to tofu, this is the place to start. The different textures offered by the grain and roast veggies are a great contrast to the fluffy whipped tofu, while the walnuts add a bit of crunch (and healthy fats, too).

FOR THE WHIPPED TOFU

14 ounces (400 g) firm tofu, pressed for 10 to 30 minutes (see page 30)

3 cloves garlic

2 tablespoons (30 ml) lemon juice

⅓ cup (80 g) tahini

2 teaspoons (10 g) Dijon mustard

¼ cup (60 ml) water

FOR SERVING

10 ounces (280 g) broccolini

1 tablespoon plus 2 teaspoons (25 ml) olive oil

⅛ teaspoon salt

⅛ teaspoon black pepper

½ cup (85 g) uncooked farro

2 cups (300 g) cherry tomatoes

2 teaspoons (10 ml) balsamic vinegar

Pinch of salt

¼ cup (30 g) walnut pieces

NUTRITIONAL ANALYSIS

SERVING SIZE: ¾ cup (180 g) whipped tofu, 1 cup (135 g) veggie/grain mixture, 2½ ounces (40 g) broccolini

PER SERVING: 437 calories; 25 g fat; 21 g protein; 30 g carbohydrates; 11 g fiber

Combine the pressed tofu, garlic, lemon juice, tahini, mustard, and water in a food processor. Process for about 3 minutes, until smooth and lightly whipped, stopping to scrape down the sides a couple times as needed. Set aside.

Preheat the oven to 425°F (220°C). Line a 18 by 13-inch (45 by 33 cm) sheet pan with parchment paper.

To make the serving vegetables and grain, toss the broccolini with 1 tablespoon (15 ml) olive oil, salt, and pepper in a large mixing bowl. Arrange evenly on the prepared pan and roast for 20 minutes, or until partially browned.

Prepare the farro according to package directions.

Heat the remaining 2 teaspoons (10 ml) olive oil in a small skillet over medium heat. Add the cherry tomatoes and cook, stirring occasionally, until bursting, 5 to 7 minutes. Add the balsamic vinegar and salt. Cook for 2 minutes more, then remove from heat.

Assemble the dish by adding ¾ cup (180 g) of the tofu mixture to each plate. Top with about 1 cup (135 g) of the veggie and grain mixture and 1 tablespoon (8 g) walnut pieces. Serve the broccolini on the side.

NOTES

- **Tip:** Whip the tofu for a little longer than you think you need to. This incorporates plenty of air into the tofu and makes it nice and fluffy.

- **Easy Swap:** If you can't find broccolini, regular broccoli florets, cut into small, bite-size pieces will work well. You may need to increase the roasting time by 5 minutes.

ZESTY QUINOA WITH BLACK BEANS AND CORN

■ **YIELD:**
6 SERVINGS

■ **PREP TIME:**
5 MINUTES

■ **COOK TIME:**
25 MINUTES

This simple, Mexican-inflected vegan recipe is packed with protein, fiber, and plenty of flavor. Together, corn and beans make a complete protein, making it a really hearty, satisfying, plant-based main dish. No lengthy shopping list required, either; it calls for cupboard staples that you're sure to have on hand.

1 cup (170 g) uncooked quinoa

1 (15-ounce/400 g) can black beans

1 (15-ounce/425 g) can no-salt-added corn

1 (10-ounce/280 g) can diced tomatoes and chiles, such as Rotel brand

1 tablespoon (6 g) ground cumin

1 teaspoon chili powder

1 teaspoon onion powder

1 teaspoon garlic powder

1 teaspoon paprika

¼ teaspoon salt

1 tablespoon (15 ml) lime juice

2 avocados, peeled, pitted, and sliced

Cook the quinoa according to package directions. Meanwhile, drain the black beans and corn and rinse well.

Place a high-sided skillet over medium heat. Add the beans, corn, and tomatoes and warm gently. Add the cumin, chili powder, onion powder, garlic powder, paprika, salt, and lime juice and stir well to combine. Add the cooked quinoa and cook for 7 minutes more.

Divide among six serving bowls, top each with avocado, and serve.

NOTES

- **Tip:** Be sure to cook the quinoa until all the liquid has evaporated and fluff with a fork for the best consistency before adding it to the bean mixture.

- **Easy Swaps:** For a milder dish, use 1½ teaspoons paprika and omit the chili powder.

NUTRITIONAL ANALYSIS

SERVING SIZE: 1½ cups (250 g)

PER SERVING: 335 calories; 10 g fat; 13 g protein; 51 g carbohydrates; 12 g fiber

INSULIN-FRIENDLY CHICKEN FRIED RICE

YIELD:
6 SERVINGS

PREP TIME:
10 MINUTES

COOK TIME:
20 MINUTES

My version of chicken fried rice puts a nutritious spin on a classic takeout favorite. Adding cauliflower rice and frozen veggies boosts fiber content without sacrificing flavor, and the result is a filling, balanced meal that satisfies cravings while supporting blood sugar balance. (Cauliflower rice is great for reducing carbs but it does change a dish's texture, so I've used half cauli-rice and half regular rice here to adjust the carb and fiber content while preserving the original texture as much as possible.)

- 2 tablespoons (30 ml) olive oil
- 2 large boneless, skinless chicken breasts, cut into 1-inch (2.5 cm) cubes
- 1 tablespoon (15 ml) toasted sesame oil
- 1 small yellow onion, diced
- 3 cloves garlic, minced
- 10 ounces (280 g) frozen peas and carrots
- 10 ounces (280 g) frozen cauliflower rice
- 3 cups (450 g) cooked jasmine rice
- 4 large eggs
- 3 to 4 tablespoons (45 to 60 ml) low-sodium soy sauce
- 1 tablespoon (15 ml) sriracha
- 2 teaspoons (10 ml) fish sauce (optional)
- 2 green onions, light and dark green parts only, thinly sliced

Heat the olive oil in a large skillet over medium heat. Add the chicken and pan fry, about 10 minutes, until it reaches an internal temperature of 165°F (75°C) and no pink remains. Cover the chicken in the skillet and set aside to keep warm.

Meanwhile, heat the sesame oil in a large wok over medium-high heat. Add the onion and garlic and saute for 3 minutes. Add the frozen peas and carrots and cauliflower rice and stir-fry for 5 minutes more. Reduce the heat to medium-low. Add the cooked rice and chicken, stirring until combined.

Push everything over to one side of the wok. Crack the eggs into the empty side, break the yolks, and stir constantly with a rubber spatula until scrambled. Mix with the rest of the ingredients.

Add the soy sauce, sriracha, and fish sauce, if using. Serve topped with the green onions.

NOTES

- **Tip:** If you're sensitive to spicy foods, add the sriracha 1 teaspoon at a time; you may not need to use the full 1 tablespoon (15 ml).

- **Easy Swaps:** Use any other frozen veggies in place of the peas and carrots. Swapping soy sauce for coconut aminos is a good way to reduce a recipe's sodium content. I chose not to use it in this recipe for the best flavor, but you can substitute it if you'd like.

NUTRITIONAL ANALYSIS

SERVING SIZE: 2 cups (450 g)

PER SERVING: 308 calories; 15 g fat; 34 g protein; 13 g carbohydrates; 5 g fiber

EGG ROLL IN A BOWL

This easy stir-fry delivers all the flavor of takeout egg rolls minus the (less healthy) fried shells. It's got ground pork for protein and premade coleslaw for a fiber boost. Plus, using fermented foods like low-sodium soy sauce helps to maintain a healthy gut. Gut health is directly related to how well you digest and absorb food, which also influences your metabolic health.

■ **YIELD:**
4 SERVINGS

■ **PREP TIME:**
10 MINUTES

■ **COOK TIME:**
5 MINUTES

■ **ASSEMBLY TIME:**
5 MINUTES

FOR THE EGG ROLL BOWLS

1 teaspoon toasted sesame oil

1 pound (450 g) ground pork

½ cup (50 g) sliced green onions, white and green parts separated

1 (14-ounce/400 g) bag tricolor coleslaw mix

3 cloves garlic, minced

2 tablespoons (30 ml) low-sodium soy sauce or coconut aminos

2 teaspoons (10 ml) rice vinegar

1 tablespoon (6 g) ground ginger

Dried red pepper flakes (optional)

Sesame seeds, for garnish

FOR THE SAUCE

¼ cup (60 g) mayonnaise

2 tablespoons (30 g) store-bought garlic chili paste

⅛ teaspoon salt

To make the egg roll bowls, heat the sesame oil in a large skillet over medium-high heat. Add the ground pork and the whites of the green onions to the pan, and cook for 5 minutes, breaking the pork apart with a wooden spoon so that it cooks evenly.

Add the remaining green parts of the green onions, coleslaw mix, garlic, soy sauce, rice vinegar, ginger, and red pepper flakes, if using. Saute for 3 to 5 minutes more, until the coleslaw is tender.

To make the sauce, whisk together the mayonnaise, garlic chili paste, and salt in a small bowl.

Divide the stir-fry mixture among four plates. Top with a generous dollop of sauce and garnish with sesame seeds.

NOTES

- **Tips:** This dish is very low in carbs. However, it's important to consume enough carbohydrates over the course of the day to improve insulin sensitivity. So, if it suits your needs, you can add ½ to 1 cup (100 to 200 g) of cooked rice to a portion for a balanced meal.

- **Easy Swaps:** Swap the ground pork with ground chicken. You can also use shredded cabbage and carrots instead of a prepared coleslaw mix.

NUTRITIONAL ANALYSIS

SERVING SIZE: 2 cups (250 g) pork and veg mixture, 2 tablespoons (30 ml) sauce

PER SERVING: 484 calories; 35 g fat; 31 g protein; 9 g carbohydrates; 3 g fiber

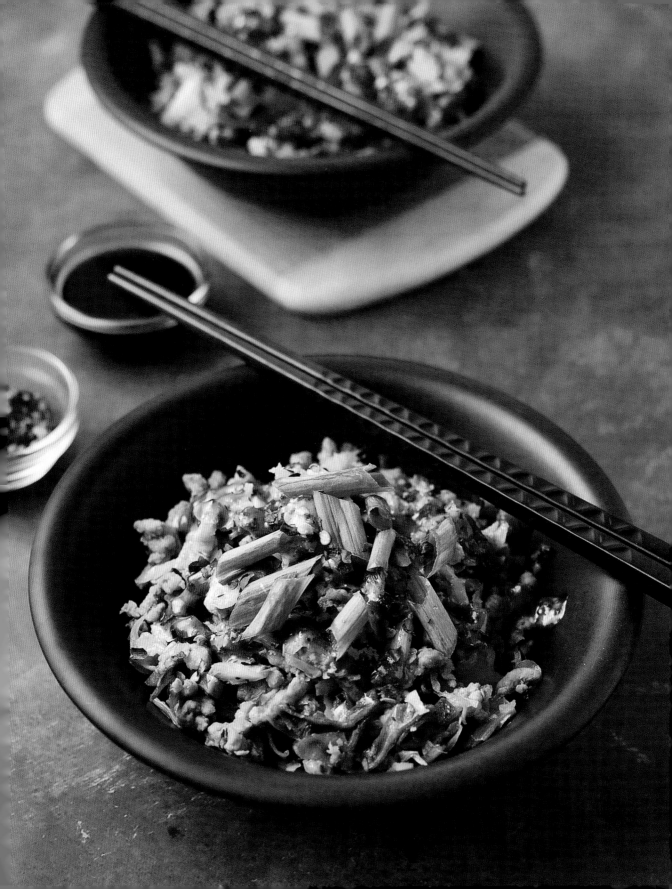

KOREAN-STYLE RICE BOWL

This bounteous rice bowl is my take on Korean bibimbap, a warming mixture of rice, vegetables, and protein. There are a few moving parts in this recipe, but don't worry—it's very simple and easy to make, and so satisfying.

YIELD:
4 SERVINGS

PREP TIME:
25 MINUTES

COOK TIME:
20 MINUTES

ASSEMBLY TIME:
5 MINUTES

14 ounces (400 g) extra-firm tofu

1 cup (185 g) uncooked basmati or jasmine rice

¼ cup (60 ml) low-sodium soy sauce

¼ cup (60 ml) coconut aminos

2 tablespoons (30 g) gochujang (chili paste)

2 tablespoons (30 ml) toasted sesame oil

1 tablespoon (15 ml) rice vinegar

2 teaspoons (4 g) ground ginger

1 tablespoon (9 g) minced garlic

2 tablespoons (30 ml) water

2 cups (180 g) broccoli florets

2 cups (160 g) whole mushrooms

2 tablespoons (30 ml) olive oil

Pinch each salt

Pinch of black pepper

10 ounces (280 g) frozen cauliflower rice

4 large eggs

1 cup (240 g) kimchi

2 medium-size avocados, peeled, pitted, and sliced

1 tablespoon (9 g) sesame seeds

Sriracha, for topping (optional)

Preheat the oven to 450°F (230°C). Line two 9½ by 13-inch (24 by 33 cm) sheet pans with parchment paper.

Press the tofu for at least 10 minutes before using (see page 30 for instructions).

Meanwhile, whisk together the soy sauce, coconut aminos, gochujang, sesame oil, rice vinegar, ginger, garlic, and 2 tablespoons (30 ml) of water in a small bowl.

Cut the pressed tofu into ¼-inch (6 mm) thick rectangular slices along the shorter side of the block. Arrange in a shallow bowl or baking dish, toss with two-thirds of the soy sauce mixture, and marinate for 10 minutes.

While the tofu is marinating, cook the basmati rice according to package directions or using a rice cooker.

Transfer the tofu onto one of the prepared baking sheets and arrange in a single layer. Discard the excess marinade. Bake for 20 minutes, flipping halfway through.

Toss the broccoli florets and mushrooms in a large bowl with the olive oil, salt, and pepper. Spread on a separate baking sheet and roast for 15 to 20 minutes, or until the florets are slightly browned.

Steam the cauliflower rice according to package directions, then stir it into the basmati or jasmine rice.

Five minutes before the tofu and vegetables are ready, apply cooking spray to a large skillet and place over medium heat; cook the eggs over easy.

To assemble the bowls, put one-quarter of the rice mixture in each one. Top each with one-quarter of the tofu, broccoli, and mushrooms. Add 1 egg, ¼ cup (40 g) kimchi, half of a sliced avocado, and a sprinkle of sesame seeds. Drizzle with sriracha, if desired.

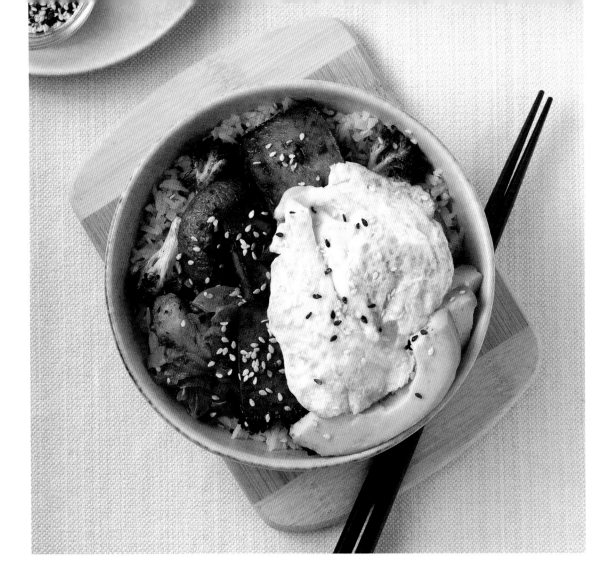

NUTRITIONAL ANALYSIS

SERVING SIZE: 4 ounces (120 g) tofu, ¾ cup (150 g) rice, 2 cups (150 g) veggies and toppings

PER SERVING: 535 calories; 36 g fat; 28 g protein; 33 g carbohydrates; 13 g fiber

NOTES

- **Tips:** You can find gochujang in the Asian aisle in your local grocery store, in an Asian market, or online. Gochujang is used in a few Asian-inspired recipes in this book and, once opened, will last in the fridge for about 1 year.

- **Easy Swaps:** Not a fan of broccoli or mushrooms? Feel free to swap them with your favorite vegetables. You can also swap the tofu with chicken, if you prefer.

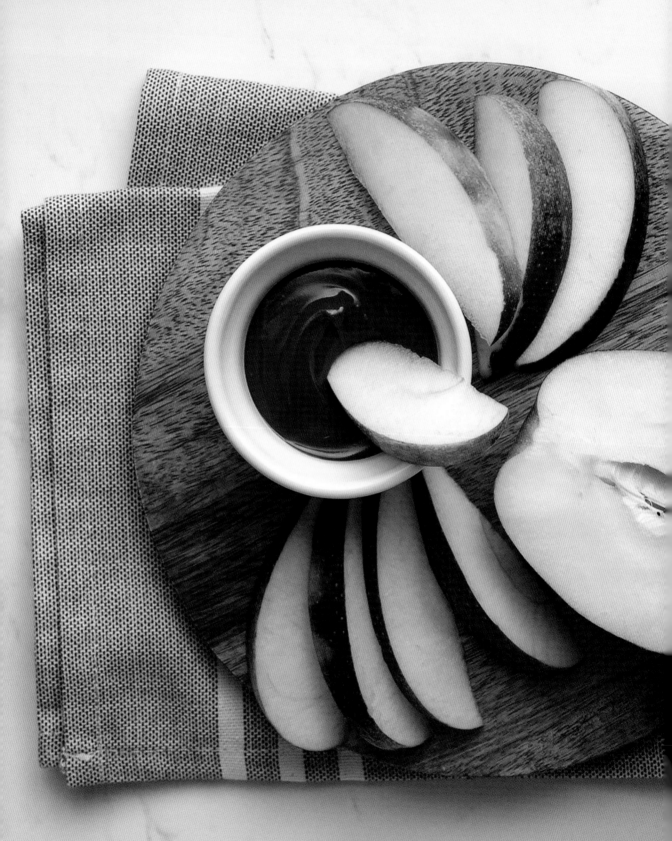

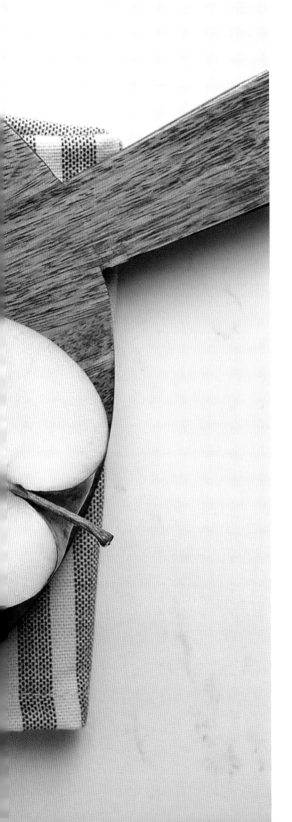

CHAPTER 6

10 Snacks and Treats in 10 Minutes

Some people can get through the day on three meals, but others need a couple of snacks throughout the day to keep up their energy levels. If that sounds like you, you'll want to choose high-fiber, high-protein options that'll see you through to your next meal without spiking your blood sugar or insulin levels. This chapter can help. It has plenty of ideas for savory snacks, and wholesome sweet treats, too. After all, enjoying desserts in moderation is good for the soul.

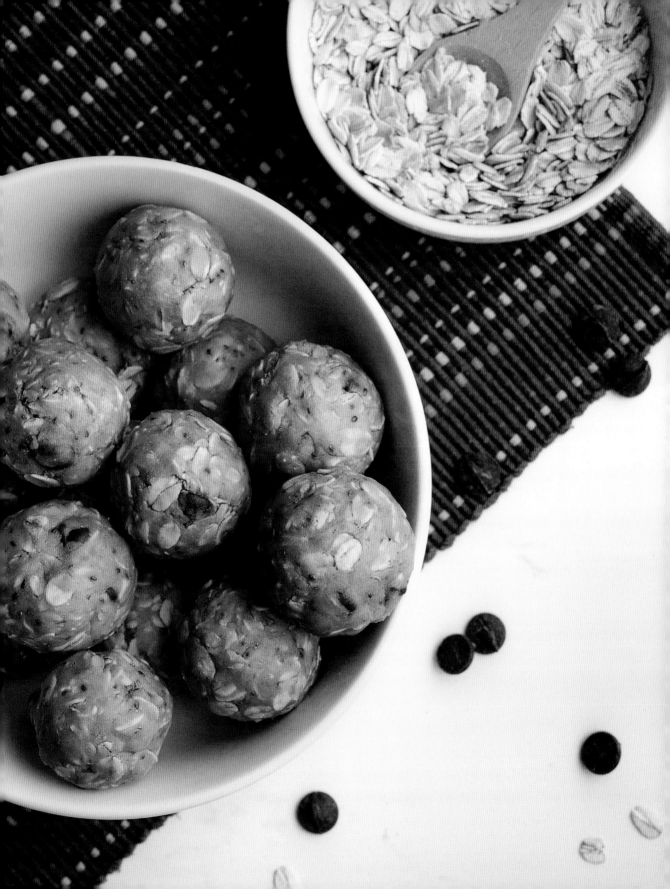

PROTEIN BALLS

⫶ **YIELD:**
6 SERVINGS

⫶ **PREP TIME:**
10 MINUTES

It's generally best to get your nutrients, including protein, from whole foods, but sometimes it's okay to use a supplement to help you to meet your daily goals. These treats are packed with protein to stave off hunger and provide lasting energy, and it's easy to make them gluten-free and vegan, too.

---

1 cup (90 g) old-fashioned oats

¾ cup (180 g) natural sugar-free peanut butter

¼ cup (30 g) vanilla protein powder

2 tablespoons (30 ml) sugar-free maple-flavored syrup

1 tablespoon (10 g) chia seeds

3 tablespoons (30 g) sugar-free chocolate chips

1 to 2 tablespoons (15 to 30 ml) water or milk, as needed

Combine the oats, peanut butter, protein powder, maple-flavored syrup, chia seeds, and chocolate chips in a mixing bowl and stir well to mix. Add the water or milk, 1 tablespoon (15 ml) at a time as needed to make the texture slightly sticky and moldable.

Using your hands, roll the mixture into approximately 12 protein balls. Store in an airtight container in the refrigerator for up to 7 days.

NOTES

- **Tip:** You might find that the batter is slightly crumbly and difficult to mix at first, but keep going—it will start to stick together as you continue to stir.
- **Easy Swaps:** Swap the chocolate chips for the same amount of coconut, raisins, or another favorite topping. Use gluten-free oats in place of regular oats, or use water instead of milk for a vegan version.

NUTRITIONAL ANALYSIS

SERVING SIZE: 2 balls

PER SERVING: 290 calories; 19 g fat; 13 g protein; 19 g carbohydrates; 6 g fiber

WHIPPED FETA DIP, THREE WAYS

YIELD:
12 SERVINGS

PREP TIME:
10 MINUTES

Paired with Greek yogurt, feta cheese creates a whipped, high-protein dip that's easy to tweak according to your (or your guests') preferences. Sweet or savory, it makes a moreish appetizer and a fabulous snack.

FOR PLAIN WHIPPED FETA DIP

- 8 ounces (225 g) feta cheese
- ⅓ cup (80 g) plain nonfat Greek yogurt
- 2 tablespoons (30 ml) avocado oil
- 2 tablespoons (30 ml) lemon juice
- 1 clove garlic, chopped
- Toppings: Sprinkle of dried red pepper flakes, pine nuts, chopped parsley, and avocado oil
- Dippers: Whole-grain or sourdough crostini, pita chips, cooled roasted carrots

TO MAKE THE PLAIN WHIPPED FETA DIP

Combine the feta cheese, yogurt, avocado oil, lemon juice, and garlic in a food processor and blend well, stopping twice to scrape down the sides of the bowl.

Transfer to a serving plate. Top with a sprinkle of dried red pepper flakes, pine nuts, and chopped parsley. Drizzle with avocado oil. Serve with the crostini, pita chips, and carrots.

FOR PUMPKIN WHIPPED FETA DIP

- 8 ounces (225 g) feta cheese
- ⅓ cup (80 g) plain nonfat Greek yogurt
- 1 cup (240 g) canned pumpkin puree
- 2 tablespoons (30 g) honey
- 2 teaspoons (2 g) fresh thyme leaves
- Toppings: Fresh thyme leaves, chopped walnuts, and honey
- Dippers: Whole-grain or sourdough crostini, cooled roasted carrots and cauliflower

TO MAKE THE PUMPKIN WHIPPED FETA DIP

Combine the feta cheese, yogurt, pumpkin, honey, and thyme in a food processor and blend well, stopping twice to scrape down the sides of the bowl.

Transfer to a serving plate. Sprinkle the thyme and walnuts on top and drizzle with honey. Serve with the crostini, carrots, and cauliflower.

FOR STRAWBERRY-BASIL WHIPPED FETA DIP

8 ounces (225 g) feta cheese

⅓ cup (80 g) plain nonfat Greek yogurt

2 tablespoons (30 ml) avocado oil

¼ teaspoon freshly ground black pepper

2 tablespoons (4 g) chopped fresh basil, plus more for topping

1 cup (150 g) coarsely chopped strawberries

1 teaspoon balsamic vinegar

2 teaspoons (10 g) honey

Dippers: Whole-grain or sourdough crostini, pita chips

TO MAKE THE STRAWBERRY-BASIL WHIPPED FETA DIP

Combine the feta, yogurt, avocado oil, black pepper, and basil in a food processor and blend well, stopping twice to scrape down the sides of the bowl.

Create a simple compote by combining the strawberries, vinegar, and honey in a small saucepan. Cook for about 6 minutes, until the strawberries soften and the honey-balsamic mixture thickens into a glaze.

Transfer the feta mixture to a serving plate. Top with the compote and additional chopped basil. Serve with crostini or pita chips.

NOTES

- **Tip:** Don't cut corners when blending. It's the secret to smooth, fluffy dips. Blend a bit longer than you think you need to. This incorporates plenty of air and ensures that the cheese and yogurt mixture is fully whipped.

- **Easy Swaps:** Use the recipe for plain feta dip to create your own flavor combinations. For example, try adding different in-season fruits, such as blueberries. Use a variety of raw and/or roasted in-season vegetables for dipping.

NUTRITIONAL ANALYSIS

SERVING SIZE: 2 tablespoons (30 g)

PER SERVING: 75 calories; 6 g fat; 3 g protein; 1 g carbohydrates; 1 g fiber

HIGH-PROTEIN CHEESE DIP WITH MARINATED TOMATOES

YIELD:
12 SERVINGS

PREP TIME:
10 MINUTES

ASSEMBLY TIME:
5 MINUTES

Cottage cheese is a powerhouse protein source and can be blended into baked goods, casseroles, and smoothies to add up to 20 grams of protein per serving. You can also add it to dips like this flavorful and protein-packed appetizer, a guaranteed hit at any party or potluck.

- 3 cups (720 g) low-fat cottage cheese
- 1 cup (150 g) feta cheese
- ¼ cup plus 1 tablespoon (75 ml) olive oil
- 2 cups (300 g) cherry tomatoes, quartered
- 2 tablespoons (10 g) finely chopped fresh parsley
- 2 tablespoons (10 g) finely chopped fresh basil
- Crostini or multigrain crackers to serve

Blend the cottage cheese, feta cheese, and ¼ cup (60 ml) olive oil in a food processor until smooth.

Mix the cherry tomatoes with the remaining 1 tablespoon (15 ml) olive oil, parsley, and basil.

Spread the cheese mixture on a rimmed plate or shallow bowl and top with the tomato mixture. Serve with crostini or multigrain crackers.

NOTES

- **Tip:** This dip can be made ahead, but it's really best eaten fresh. I recommend making it within an hour of serving.

- **Easy Swaps:** Any variety of fresh tomatoes will work well here. In a pinch, you can also use drained sun-dried tomatoes packed in oil.

NUTRITIONAL ANALYSIS

SERVING SIZE: ½ cup (160 g) dip

PER SERVING: 125 calories; 9 g fat; 8 g protein; 3 g carbohydrates; 1 g fiber

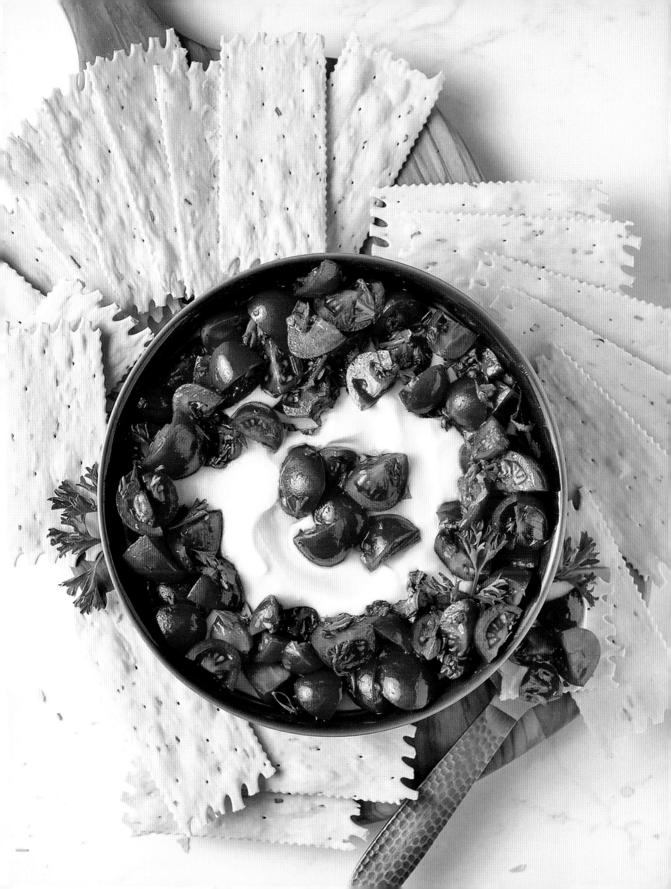

COTTAGE CHEESE CAPRESE

YIELD:
1 SERVING

PREP TIME:
5 MINUTES

You'll look forward to your afternoon snack when this elevated twist on cottage cheese is on the menu. The protein in the cottage cheese plus the fiber in the cherry tomatoes makes it a well-balanced snack, and the vinegar and basil give it a powerful punch of flavor. If you need extra carbs, add a handful of whole-grain crackers.

½ cup (120 g) low-fat cottage cheese

4 cherry tomatoes, halved

¼ teaspoon olive oil

¼ teaspoon balsamic vinegar

2 basil leaves, chopped

Flaky sea salt

Put the cottage cheese in a bowl. Add the cherry tomatoes and top with chopped basil. Drizzle with the olive oil and balsamic vinegar and add a small pinch of flaky salt.

NOTES

- **Tip:** Don't like the texture of cottage cheese? Try blending it into a creamy version. Simply add it to a food processor and pulse for 10 to 20 seconds until it reaches a smooth consistency.

- **Easy Swaps:** Replace the balsamic vinegar with a balsamic glaze (reduced balsamic vinegar) or with your favorite type of vinegar.

NUTRITIONAL ANALYSIS

SERVING SIZE: ½ cup (120 g)

PER SERVING: 120 calories; 4 g fat; 12 g protein; 6 g carbohydrates; 1 g fiber

MIX-AND-MATCH SNACK BOX

▌ YIELD:
1 SERVING

▌ ASSEMBLY TIME:
5 MINUTES

If you need suggestions for simple, blood sugar–stabilizing snacks that won't spike your insulin levels, you've come to the right place. This guided mix-and-match "recipe" will give you snack ideas for months. Just remember, balance is everything. If you need more information on pairing foods properly, check out the resources at www.megankoehn.com.

PROTEIN (PICK 1):
2 OUNCES (55 G)

Cheese cubes

Flavored tuna pack

Edamame

Any nuts of your choice (see Tip)

Flavored almonds

Crispy chickpeas

Hummus

Yogurt-based dip (read the nutrition label and choose one that's low in sugar)

Natural sugar-free peanut butter

VEGETABLE (PICK 1 TO 2):
½ CUP (ABOUT 75 G)

Cherry tomatoes

Carrots

Celery

Cauliflower

Bell peppers

Radishes

Cucumbers

FRUIT OR STARCH (PICK 1):
1 CUP (WEIGHT VARIES)

Grapes

Plum

Orange

Berries

½ banana

Whole-grain crackers

Corn tortilla chips

Choose your favorite options from the lists to the left, or use your own favorites, and add to a meal prep container or plate. Make sure to select an option from each category, remembering that foods that increase insulin sensitivity are high in fiber and protein and low in added sugar, sodium, and saturated fat. Enjoy.

NOTES

- **Tips:** If you select nuts as your protein source for this snack, consider choosing an unsalted or lower-sodium option, such as raw, unsalted cashews or almonds. (That's not to say that salted nuts are totally off-menu; just choose the option that's right for you, depending on your overall sodium consumption for the day.)

- **Easy Swaps:** There are millions of healthy foods in this world, so the lists above are incomplete. Add your own faves to these lists and cross off the foods that don't do it for you. Consider this your own personal snack list.

NUTRITIONAL ANALYSIS

SERVING SIZE: 1 snack box, varies

PER SERVING: varies

AVOCADO FETA PARTY DIP

YIELD:
6 SERVINGS

PREP TIME:
10 MINUTES

CHILL TIME:
6 HOURS

This deconstructed, sophisticated take on guacamole gets added heft from tangy feta cheese and extra flavor from fresh herbs, making it the life of the party. Corn chips are good for dipping here because they contain fiber and only a moderate amount of sodium. Choose brands that are baked rather than fried, or brands that are fried but with lower saturated fat levels (read the nutrition label); they'll be less greasy.

1 avocado, peeled, pitted, and diced

2 Roma tomatoes, chopped

¼ cup (40 g) chopped red onion

1 clove garlic, minced

1 tablespoon (15 ml) avocado oil

1 tablespoon (15 ml) red wine vinegar

1 tablespoon (3 g) chopped fresh parsley

1 tablespoon (3 g) chopped fresh oregano

4 ounces (115 g) feta cheese, crumbled

Corn chips or thickly sliced bell peppers, to serve

Put the avocado in a mixing bowl. Gently stir in the tomatoes, onion, and garlic. Add the oil, vinegar, parsley, and oregano and stir gently. Finally, add the feta and stir gently again. Cover and chill for 6 hours or overnight.

Serve with corn chips or bell pepper slices.

NOTES

- **Tips:** This dip is best prepared ahead of time. Leave it in the fridge overnight so the flavors meld. The acid in the vinegar will keep the avocado from browning, so don't worry: It will stay looking fresh.

- **Easy Swap:** Dried herbs will also work here. Use half the recommended fresh herb measurement.

NUTRITIONAL ANALYSIS

SERVING SIZE: ½ cup (90 g) dip

PER SERVING: 120 calories; 10 g fat; 4 g protein; 4 g carbohydrates; 2 g fiber

POPCORN, THREE WAYS

Popcorn is the perfect snack—filling, crunchy, and fiber-rich. It even has some protein! Skip the buttery topping and try these flavorful, healthier twists instead.

▥ YIELD:
2 SERVINGS

▥ PREP TIME:
5 MINUTES

◉ COOK TIME:
2 TO 3 MINUTES

FOR THE POPCORN

¼ cup (40 g) popcorn kernels

1 tablespoon (15 ml) olive oil (optional)

FOR VEGAN CHEESE POPCORN

¼ cup (15 g) nutritional yeast

¼ teaspoon flaky sea salt

FOR SEA SALT AND DARK CHOCOLATE POPCORN

2 tablespoons (28 g) sugar-free dark chocolate chips, melted

¼ teaspoon sea salt

FOR SAVORY HERBED POPCORN

2 tablespoons (30 ml) avocado oil (added during popping, in place of olive oil)

½ teaspoon dried oregano

½ teaspoon dried basil

½ teaspoon dried thyme

½ teaspoon garlic powder

½ teaspoon onion powder

½ teaspoon salt, or more as needed

¼ teaspoon black pepper

NUTRITIONAL ANALYSIS

SERVING SIZE: 3 cups (40 g)

PER SERVING: 140 calories; 8 g fat; 2 g protein; 20 g carbohydrates; 5 g fiber

Microwave the popcorn kernels in a covered glass bowl for 2 to 3 minutes until the popping slows. Alternatively, pop on the stovetop: Heat 1 tablespoon (15 ml) olive oil in a large pot over medium-high, add the kernels, cover, and shake until the popping slows.

To make vegan cheese popcorn, combine the nutritional yeast and salt in a small bowl. Sprinkle over the hot popcorn and stir or shake well to coat.

To make the sea salt and dark chocolate popcorn, spread the popcorn out on a 9½ by 13-inch (24 by 33 cm) sheet pan lined with parchment paper. Drizzle the melted chocolate over the popcorn and sprinkle with sea salt. Let sit for 10 minutes to harden.

To make the savory herbed popcorn, pop the kernels in avocado oil for better herb adhesion. Combine the oregano, basil, thyme, garlic powder, onion powder, salt, and pepper. Sprinkle over the hot popcorn, stir to coat, and adjust salt to taste.

Enjoy hot and fresh!

NOTES

- **Tips:** I use a Colonel Popper, a silicone bowl with a lid that makes it easy to microwave popcorn kernels without adding oil. To help your chosen flavoring stick to the popcorn, consider misting the popcorn lightly with olive oil or lightly spraying with cooking spray.

- **Easy Swaps:** Experimenting with popcorn flavors is so much fun. Mix in your favorite spices or herbs, or opt for a hint of sweetness by sprinkling it with ½ teaspoon ground cinnamon and ½ teaspoon white sugar or sugar substitute. You can create endless flavor combinations.

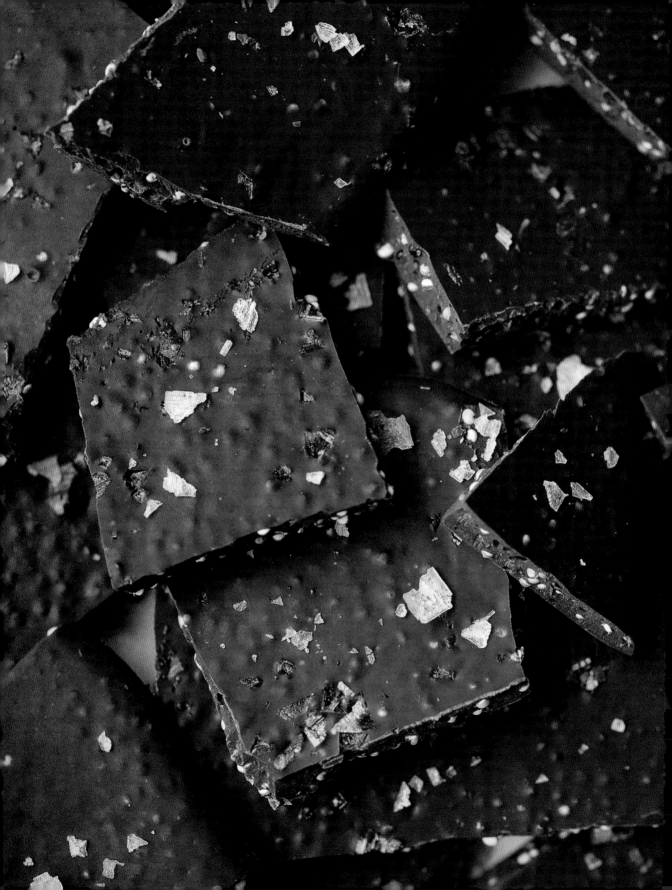

PUFFED QUINOA BARK

Quinoa is high in protein and fiber, making it a great blood-sugar stabilizer. Add it to chocolate and you'll fall in love. This sweet crispy treat is a hit in my house. It's fast and easy to make, and the combination of sweet, salty, and crunchy is so satisfying.

▥ **YIELD:**
8 SERVINGS

▥ **PREP TIME:**
10 MINUTES

▥ **CHILL TIME:**
2 HOURS

⅓ cup (60 g) uncooked quinoa

8 ounces (225 g) 75% dark chocolate

Flaky sea salt

First, puff the quinoa. Heat a small skillet over medium high heat. Once hot, add the dry quinoa. When you hear the quinoa start to pop (about 2 minutes after adding to the heat), shake often. When it is popping nonstop (about 4 minutes later), remove from the heat and shake continuously for about 1 minute. Transfer to a bowl.

Melt the chocolate in a double boiler or in the microwave in 30-second increments until melted.

Line a 9½ by 13-inch (24 by 33 cm) sheet pan with parchment paper. Fold the quinoa into the chocolate and spread evenly on the lined baking sheet until it's about ¼ to ½ inch (6 mm to 1 cm) thick.

Sprinkle flaky salt on the top and chill in the freezer for 2 hours to firm up. Break into 3-inch (7.6–cm) squares and serve.

NOTES

- **Tip:** Quinoa can burn quickly, so don't get distracted: Keep an eye on it the whole time.

- **Easy Swaps:** You can further reduce the sugar content by using 85% or 90% dark chocolate, though I think 75% dark chocolate hits the mark on this lightly sweet, low–carbohydrate dessert.

NUTRITIONAL ANALYSIS

SERVING SIZE: 1½ ounces (35 g)

PER SERVING: 165 calories; 12 g fat; 4 g protein; 13 g carbohydrates; 4 g fiber

TWO-INGREDIENT PEANUT BUTTER CHOCOLATE DIP

YIELD:
1 SERVING

PREP TIME:
5 MINUTES

It's important to work sweet treats into your regular eating pattern. This might sound surprising coming from a dietitian, but it's true. No eating pattern is sustainable if it involves cutting out your favorite foods, and that includes chocolate. This luscious dip contains protein, fiber, good fats, and no added sugar, so it'll satisfy your sweet tooth while stabilizing your blood sugar and insulin levels. The perfect treat.

2 tablespoons (30 g) natural sugar-free peanut butter

1 tablespoon (15 g) sugar-free chocolate chips

Apple slices or strawberries, for serving

Combine the peanut butter and chocolate chips to a small bowl. Microwave for 20 seconds, stir, and serve with apple slices or strawberries for dipping.

NOTES

- **Tips:** I love to dunk apple slices in this dip, but it's also wonderful drizzled over a banana or, even better, frozen over a sliced banana.

- **Easy Swaps:** Crunchy or creamy peanut butter both work fine here. You pick.

NUTRITIONAL ANALYSIS

SERVING SIZE: 3 tablespoons (45 g) dip

PER SERVING: 250 calories; 20 g fat; 8 g protein; 14 g carbohydrates; 7 g fiber

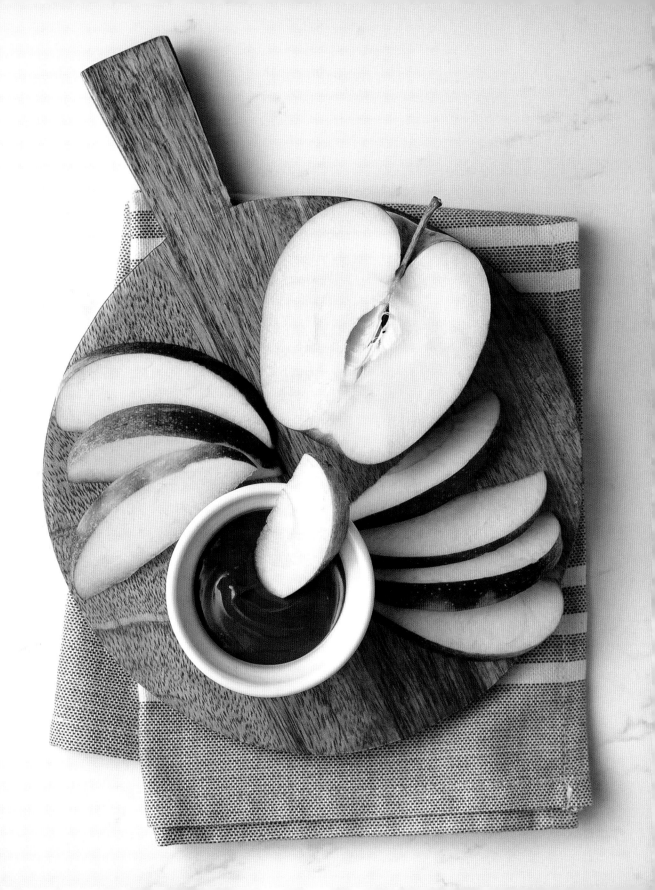

MEGAN'S EDIBLE CHOCOLATE CHIP COOKIE DOUGH

YIELD:
12 SERVINGS

PREP TIME:
10 MINUTES

I have a fond childhood memory of making a whole batch of cookie dough with my dad and siblings while my mom was away on a work trip. We didn't bake a single cookie; we just enjoyed the dough all week. Talk about rebellion! I'm no less obsessed with cookie dough now that I'm an adult, so I created a healthier version with less sugar, more fiber, and even some protein.

2 cups (180 g) old-fashioned oats

1 cup (164 g) canned chickpeas, drained and rinsed

⅓ cup (80 ml) 2% low-fat milk

¼ cup (50 g) white sugar baking blend substitute

¼ cup (48 g) brown sugar baking blend substitute

½ teaspoon salt

½ teaspoon pure vanilla extract

2 tablespoons plus 1 teaspoon (35 ml) melted coconut oil

½ cup (85 g) sugar-free chocolate chips

Put the oats in a single-serve blender and blend for about 10 seconds, until a fine flour is formed. Set aside in a small bowl.

Add the chickpeas and milk to the blender and blend for about 20 seconds or until smooth, stopping once to scrape down the sides. Use a rubber spatula to transfer to a large mixing bowl.

Add both sugar substitutes, salt, vanilla, and melted coconut oil. Using a hand mixer, mix until combined. Add the oat flour, ½ cup (45 g) at a time, continuing to mix until well combined. Gently fold in the chocolate chips.

Serve immediately or refrigerate. The cookie dough will stay fresh in an airtight container in the fridge for 4 days, or in the freezer for up to 6 months.

NUTRITIONAL ANALYSIS

SERVING SIZE: ¼ cup (85 g)

PER SERVING: 130 calories; 5 g fat; 3 g protein; 20 g carbohydrates; 4 g fiber

NOTES

- **Tips:** I like to use a single-serve blender for easy clean up, but if you don't have one, a food processor will work just as well.

- **Easy Swaps:** If you're not a fan of chocolate chips, try other mix-ins in the same amount, such as raisins, nuts, or a tablespoon of coconut flakes.

Acknowledgments

I'd like to thank my husband, Maxwell, for being my primary taste tester, my biggest cheerleader, and my constant source of support. A special thanks to my mom, dad, and all my friends who joined me in recipe testing along the way.

To my grandparents, Denny and Susie: Your unwavering belief in me has been a lifelong gift. Your encouragement and pride fuel my ambition to keep growing and helping as many people as possible.

I'm deeply grateful to my clients, who make my work so fulfilling.

Finally, a huge thank you to the Quarto team for bringing this book to life and helping countless people with insulin resistance and metabolic conditions thrive.

About the Author

Megan Koehn, RDN, is a registered dietitian nutritionist, the founder of the Drop Diabetes Program, and a certified nutrition counselor dedicated to helping individuals manage type 2 diabetes and prediabetes. After having worked as a diabetes dietitian in outpatient care for more than three years, Megan recognized the gaps in diabetes support and created the Drop Diabetes Program to bridge them. Since launching the program in 2020, she has helped more than 800 clients achieve better health and has culti-vated a strong following of more than 200,000 across social media platforms. Her expertise has been featured in major publications, including *Newsweek* and MSN.

In her free time she enjoys exploring the mountains or discovering new eateries with her husband, Maxwell.

You can find her on all social media platforms as @Type2DiabetesCoachMegan. Visit her website at www.megankoehn.com.

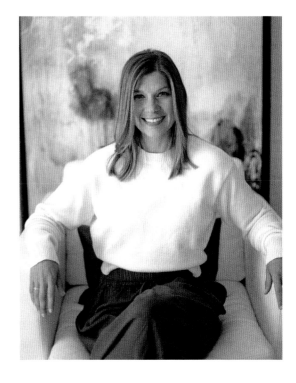

Index